PENGUIN BOOKS
MOVE BETTER

Shikha Puri Arora is a rehab and movement coach. She has written articles on posture and pain-free living for the *Free Press Journal*, and is certified in various levels of rehab training (Australia), therapeutic yoga, Pilates and rolfing. Shikha has experience for over a decade in treating individuals with various musculoskeletal issues—fibromyalgia, scoliosis, kyphosis, ankylosing spondylitis, arthritis, herniated and slipped discs, frozen shoulders, and knee and hip replacements. Her expertise also extends to individuals who suffer from cancer, asthma and other respiratory ailments. She is the founder of Move Better Wellness, which is the first online and offline rehab fitness platform in India that offers one-on-one rehab fitness sessions, myofascial release massages, performance nutrition services, wellness courses and corporate wellness programmes, all under one roof.

Celebrating 35 Years of
Penguin Random House India

MOVE BETTER

A TWO-STEP GUIDE TO EFFICIENT POSTURE AND INCREASED MOBILITY

SHIKHA PURI ARORA

PENGUIN BOOKS

An imprint of Penguin Random House

PENGUIN BOOKS

USA | Canada | UK | Ireland | Australia
New Zealand | India | South Africa | China | Singapore

Penguin Books is part of the Penguin Random House group of companies
whose addresses can be found at global.penguinrandomhouse.com

Published by Penguin Random House India Pvt. Ltd
4th Floor, Capital Tower 1, MG Road,
Gurugram 122 002, Haryana, India

First published in Penguin Books by Penguin Random House India 2023

Copyright © Shikha Puri Arora 2023

Illustrations by Parthika Immaneni

All rights reserved

10 9 8 7 6 5 4 3 2 1

ISBN 9780143458142

Typeset in Minion Pro by Manipal Technologies Limited, Manipal

www.penguin.co.in

To the millions of people who have resigned themselves to the fate of injuries, aches, pains, weight gain and surgery. May this education bring peace, good health and hope!

Contents

Preface

If you're a lover of stories, you will love to do what I do. My typical day starts with someone telling me a story like this: 'I am a very active person, and I have always been blessed with good health. But a few years ago, I developed this intense knee pain, in spite of doing yoga and walking regularly—I just don't know how! Suddenly, after a year, I developed back pain, I just don't know why! The orthopaedic doctor said it is due to my weak core. These pains reoccur at least thrice every year and I have to go back to the physiotherapist every time. Even after doing my physiotherapy exercises religiously, I still haven't found the guts to restart yoga. Many people have told me to stop sitting on the floor, but I am only 50 years old! What has happened to me suddenly? I was okay all these years! I have been doing well of late, but today my other knee is hurting, I just don't know why!'

Wherever I go and everywhere I look, someone is enacting this story. 'Oh God!!! It will take me five minutes to get up

from this sofa! My hip is locked and my back is jammed . . .
Help! Please lend me a hand . . . Don't just leave me here and go!'

How many times have we seen and heard this story?

A true story of a 30-year-old I met a few years ago: 'Hi! I
have come to you today because my main goal for this year is
to have enough mobility so I can get my legs into my pants
and not get stuck while I pull them up.'

'I am 19, my knees are 41, my shoulders are 54 and my
back turns 72 tomorrow.' Sarcasm like this is seen all over
social media, but in truth, it is the sorry plight of the youth
and global population today.

After all these years, I feel there are no new stories left, as
everyone has a similar one. Here is mine . . . In my twenties, I
had a severe bout of unsteadiness that persisted for a month.
I ran to various doctors and medical specialists, getting
all possible tests done. There was no concrete diagnosis, as
nothing showed up in the test reports. Most of the consulting
doctors said, 'Child, there is nothing wrong with you. There
are people with worse degeneration. Go home!' I was fed up—
the cause of my symptoms was escaping medical detection and
did not have a remedy. As a few years went by, I developed
other aches and pains. Despite availing local remedies, they
would appear and disappear, only for similar ones or others
to show up.

Today, many individuals, young and old, struggle to find
solutions for untimely pain, migraines, vertigo, false heart
pain, breathlessness, lack of mobility, chronic fatigue and
early degeneration without permanent remedies. One can
google a lot of information today, but it is usually vague and
doesn't troubleshoot an individual's specific issues. Thus, it is
mostly misleading.

While seeking the cause and a permanent cure for my neck pain, shoulder pain, back pain, foot pain and knee pain, I discovered that these aches are *symptoms* and not the actual *problem*. Their origin lies in our faulty mechanics. The cause and cure of these symptoms are rooted in our lifestyle. Our movement patterns, lifestyle habits, postures, breathing habits, hobbies and our unenlightened approach to ergonomics contribute largely to the dysfunction that we experience as symptoms.

To ease my own health and decrease the probability of recurring aches and pains, I travelled all over the world, trying to learn different modalities of fitness-based techniques as well as clinical approaches to treating musculoskeletal* health problems. To my surprise, I found that most of these symptoms that are a nuisance and may even seem life-threatening and debilitating can be cured at home with the right knowledge. The 'Move Better Course' outlined in this book is designed to make you pain-free for life within ten days.

Our mastery in using the body efficiently largely impacts our overall health and well-being. Our goal should be to improve our movement skills. Instead of doing this, some choose easier but temporary solutions and cures, such as popping a painkiller. Had I been content with easier and less time-consuming solutions, not only would I have added more musculoskeletal problems every year to my list, but my health on all fronts would have deteriorated altogether.

---

* Musculoskeletal problems are injuries or disorders of the muscles, nerves, joints, tendons and spinal discs. A sprain or strain, tear, back pain and other pains, osteoarthritis, tendinitis, fractures or arthritis are some examples.

Without a commitment towards functioning with better biomechanics,* I would have blamed my issues on age and might have developed the 'poor me' attitude or the 'why me?' belief. *Our ill-health and pain adversely shape our mental attitudes and have the capacity to impact self-efficacy, confidence and create significant psychological stress and behavioural changes.*

Niggling aches, pains and discomfort affect the brain and reduce our output at work by 20 per cent! Think of the amount of money we lose with a 20 per cent reduction in mental output! We don't add this to the list of our expenses and medical bills. Tiny aches and pains are disguised financial costs that go unaccounted for, for years and years.

> While the prevalence of musculoskeletal conditions increases with age, younger people are also affected, often during their peak income-earning years. The societal impact of early retirement in terms of direct health-care costs and indirect (i.e., work absenteeism or productivity loss) costs is enormous. Reduced ability to work leads to early retirement, lower levels of well-being and reduced ability to participate in society.[1]—WHO

I have even experienced my own dentist quitting her practice after so many years of slogging in medical school, because of a slipped disc. Professional life goes for a toss with a single disability. While medical technology has been promising enough to push life expectancy from 53 years to 90 years,[2] our

---

* The mechanics of our body in locomotion or exercise. The study of our movement loads, motion, stress and strain on the body's movement, size, shape and structure.

work life is becoming shorter. Our grandfathers worked for 40 years, fathers 33 years and now, the newer generation works for merely 25 years, as health issues and the inability to cope with work pressures lead to early retirement. Even though life expectancy has increased, quality of health continues to decline. *This is why there is a need to have a solution that isn't only focused on increasing life expectancy or making the body more comfortable, but one that adds to the quality of life we lead while enjoying the journey.*

Musculoskeletal problems are very similar to many other lifestyle diseases. Just as too much sugar, starch or fat manifests later as diabetes and heart disease, faulty movement patterns surface someday as chronic pain. This is why it is about time the average Indian prioritizes quality of movement and posture, realizing their importance because, like all other lifestyle diseases, musculoskeletal problems also pave the way to hell.

Living at the peak of our well-being is the birthright of every individual. This book brings forth the solutions that serve to eradicate most musculoskeletal problems and symptoms arising from them. Movement education is beneficial for all ages, as it increases physical efficiency while decreasing the risk of injury and pain. For more than a decade, I have helped thousands of people, including children as young as 8 years and seniors in their 80s, to change their lives from *dis-ease* to complete ease, with optimized well-being and performance. I am excited to share my methods of transformation, to empower eager individuals who are motivated to:

- stay pain-free with no recurring musculoskeletal dysfunction;

- move better with skill so you can move more with ease and efficiency;
- safely add more movement to life;
- improve brain activity and mental health for children and adults;
- have better health in the case of the elderly;
- delay or avert surgery;
- control and manage the effects of genetic predispositions;
- maintain ideal weight;
- improve ergonomics and become more efficient at the workplace.

This book encompasses tried-and-tested solutions used worldwide in many clinical and fitness set-ups. These skills are applied by millions of sports physiotherapists, high-performance coaches, posturologists, biomechanists, myofascial therapists and alternative healing coaches.

I welcome you to the world of 'Move Better Wellness' (www.movebetterwellness.in), which is India's first rehab fitness platform for all ages, fitness and health levels. We specialize in customizing courses and sessions that focus on movement reconditioning, restoration and rehabilitation *within your fitness sessions* to help you save time and money. By introducing these revolutionary methods, my vision is to empower individuals and bring better health and well-being to our society for generations to come. I wish you tons of luck on your movement-health journey and I am always here to support you.

Shikha Puri Arora
Kemps Corner, Mumbai
Email: shikha@movebetterwellness.in

Introduction

Exercise today is promoted by motivating one towards a sense of purpose or goal—losing weight, achieving better looks, minimizing the risk of health problems, grabbing the best marriage proposals. For parents, exercise means getting their kids enrolled in some sport or the other just because other kids are doing it. *Unfortunately, movement isn't considered a natural way of life any more.* Our ancestors did not have cars, so walking or cycling for daily errands was not purpose driven but very much a natural part of life. I remember with immense pleasure the occasional days when I walked back home after school with friends instead of taking the school bus. That was considered fun! There are other types of purpose-driven movement, like walking the four *dhaams*, circumambulation of holy shrines and waiting in long queues in the heat for *darshan* of our favourite idol—I call this the 'religious workout'. All the effort and sweat are worth it because it is purpose driven. But when it comes to minor things, such as passing the salt across the table, it is considered a task. 'I have worked hard all day . . . pass the remote . . . and get me water . . . and some food . . . and a towel . . .'

Here's the catch: you got out of bed, sat down for breakfast, sat in your vehicle to go to work, sat in the office, sat on the way back home and sat after coming home, claiming you have worked hard and don't wish to move. Once home, everything is too much of an effort. The average Indian feels movement in daily life isn't pleasurable.

What are my beliefs about movement? Is it a way of life or simply a chore? Am I confusing movement with purpose or exercise? Most feel movement drains their energy and avoiding it brings comfort. Others consider only exercise as movement. But we are moving throughout our day even when not exercising. Do babies move and play or do they exercise? They climb, roll and run all day without counting the number of squats and clocking the time they completed it in. I wonder when the invention of a rest day or holiday began to mean *no* movement! We can't take breaks from movement. The human body was designed to move and be in action. Movement is who we are and what we do. Movement and activity are nature's way of facilitating creation and dissolution, a matrix of energy. Energy is life. The ancient yogis called this energy, or the vital force, *Praanaa*. Existence is Praanaa and Praanaa is present in the animate and inanimate. When observed under a microscope, even non-living entities show movement of cells. Energy is the vital force that governs us, so we can't say we are out of energy and can't move. If one is out of energy, it means that their internal biology and physiology is dis-eased. Well-being is seen in bodies that align with nature's innate harmony. Disease is moving against it. Movement is like the flowing rivers—idleness is akin to smelly, stagnant waters. We find ourselves complaining and not in unity with our environment only when our mind, movement and rest are completely out of sync. An example of this is the increased number of musculoskeletal problems we saw in people during the COVID-19 pandemic. Most people I treated complained of pain because of being home-bound. When the environment we are thrown into decides the fate of our health, we have to understand that something isn't in sync. *The environment is an extension of our body and movement is what unifies us with our environment to make us one.*

If we could see cells move, we would notice that nature is all about grace, poise, flexibility, balance and constant activity. The body is part of nature, made of five elements—earth, water, fire, air and space. *Being in sync with the universe is being alive, alert, in motion and balancing movement with rest, as is the case in the galaxy and the animal kingdom.* If movement is not a priority and requires effort, then dis-ease becomes our disconnection with movement. When we question our relationship with movement, are we also questioning our very existence, our Praanaa? *The sign of the Life Principle* within us is movement.*

One of my favourite quotes from the Gospel of Thomas reads,

> Jesus says: 'If people ask you: "Where have you come from?" tell them: "I have come from Light."

---

* The vital force or animating principle by which all organs inside the body function and by which all forces in the universe work. When Praanaa abandons any living body, it is said to be dead.

'If someone says to you: "Who are you?" say: "I am the offspring of the Living Father."

'If people ask you: "What is the sign of your Father within you?" Tell them: "IT IS MOVEMENT AND REST [emphasis added]."'

1

Moving Better before Moving More

It is believed that first impressions are usually the last ones. The way we move, sit, stand, walk and carry ourselves is the first impression that reveals good, average or poor health. Some individuals think that if they can move a lot, they are healthy and fit. But despite the ability to lift heavy weights, or walk and run 25–50 kilometres, or be very committed to a fitness routine or new-year fitness goals, most individuals still experience some degree of muscular discomfort, spasms and sprains through the day which are ignored. Enduring aches and pains is considered 'normal' for some time till one cannot sustain the latest fitness fads that have become too challenging to continue.

There are others who may try to add some movement to their daily lives because the doctor prescribed it. Walking is considered the safest for the average out-of-shape individual. The 'walking to lose weight' prescription may help keep one's weight in check and can also improve the blood tests that were out of the ordinary range. For some, even if their legs and feet get tired and swollen, they see no option but to push past certain aches and pains to meet their health goals. But once those health goals are achieved, these individuals with average fitness fall out of their routine as they feel moving is a form of drudgery. Individuals think that not moving is a sign of laziness and procrastination or dislike for exercise. But in truth, it is none of these! Walking and moving just doesn't feel easy for most. This is because a sedentary individual's basic movement functions have already become inhibited. So, even simple movements like walking are not sustainable measures to achieve health goals. One must not erroneously assume that attempts to regain fitness, lose weight or become more active suddenly adopted as a goal will make one better as time goes by.

Whether one exercises because one is passionate about it or because the doctor asked them to, does the exercise routine come with an assurance that it will prevent aches and pains, future surgery, injury and degeneration? Most of us mistakenly assume 'yes' because we are attempting to move more.

> It is not how much or how little you do, but how *efficiently* and *easily* you do it over a sustained period of time, free of aches and pains.

Feeling Good or Feeling Healthy

I often ask people how they feel after exercising. Many will claim that they feel good during and after their exercise routines. But are we defining feeling good as the psychological satisfaction we get on completing a healthy goal every day? We need to reassess the true meaning of feeling good and good health. *Feeling good should come from feeling mobile and pain-free in all our movements through the day.* Good health isn't simply denoted by claims such as 'my cholesterol, diabetes and high blood pressure are now under control', or 'I have lost weight' or 'I exercise so I am leading a healthy life'.

We may feel good after exercising, but most of us feel a decline in our fitness levels and health over the years as we are unable to get up from a chair or out of the car after a long drive without dealing with a stiff back, a limp in the leg or a nagging neck pain. At some point in our lives, having been rendered sedentary by an illness, we might have felt like our whole body was jammed and moving may have felt like the daily ordeal our grandparents face. 'Oh my! I feel like an old person! I think I'm ageing!' is an exclamation often uttered by the young twenty- or thirty-year-olds on returning to fitness after an illness. It can be the same feeling for a frequent traveller who is glued to the airplane or car seat for hours on end. In all these experiences, where our immediate environment results in less movement, the long-term repercussion is our restricted ability of movement. *Mobility is not about our age, being 'born flexible' or being able to meet our occupational demands. Instead, mobility is a 'choice' we need to make every day.* Every morning we should feel excited to move and be mobile, just as we felt when we were children, despite the challenges our environment throws at us at any age.

Good health is the freedom to move in and through life despite the environmental stress and strains we are exposed to in our sedentary cultures! Good health is the feeling of freedom as our entire body works to its maximum efficiency in all our movements through the day, pain-free!

Use It—or Else You Will Lose It!

The basic problem of increasing aches and pain in daily life is due to the inferior quality of basic movement skill. This problem is unfortunately faced by a large number of people across the world. The foremost reason for this is *sedentariness.*

We have gone through a global pandemic, but how many of us are aware of the global epidemic of physical inactivity, which is associated with 5.3 million deaths a year,[1] much before the COVID-19 pandemic? The first challenge that an individual faces for regular movement is the sedentary time their occupation demands—those hours lead to inactive muscles. People say they can't feel their bum while performing a simple glute squeeze. Why don't you put down your phone and give it a try?

- Stand with your feet hip-width apart or wider.
- You can turn your feet out if you like.
- Squeeze the buttocks. In order to do so, you will tilt your pelvis to tuck your tailbone inward when you squeeze.

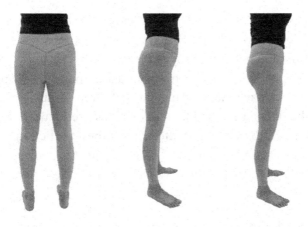

Can you feel your whole buttock when you squeeze it? Or just parts of it? 'Glute amnesia' is not uncommon and the majority of the global population faces this loss of function as unused muscles are switched off by the brain. The glutes are the largest muscles in the body and help carry loads for long periods on the legs. Imagine having them totally switched off! How efficient can we be in such a situation? How long are we going to be able to move with the added load and stress on smaller muscles, such as the quadriceps, calves and feet? These can't sustain such a burden for long hours and get tight and overused—then the pain sets in. Our movement becomes inefficient and tough beyond measure because one muscle is on a permanent holiday! This is why people feel walking is tiring and choose the easier option of hiring a cab everywhere, even if it means spending hard-earned money. *Thus, building skill and mobility in all our movements through the day is key.*

Rounded shoulders make the postural muscles of the back totally inactive, as they are in a constantly stretched-out position. While trying out activation exercises, most individuals have told me they felt those back muscles for the first time and never even knew they existed!

Even if we don't suffer from any aches and pains, we need to see if we have the full range of motion in all our joints. If our shoulders, neck, ankles, back or knees feel stuck, even if it is a mere 10 per cent, it affects our fitness output, just like pain affects our mental output. *When you start moving with an existing limitation, you only aggravate existing dysfunctions in the body.*

One cannot move more and achieve health goals with limited mobility and inactive muscles. The outcome will be pain and aggravation of muscular dysfunctions.

Our Sitting Can Influence Our Moving

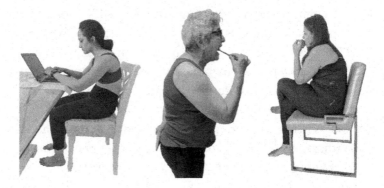

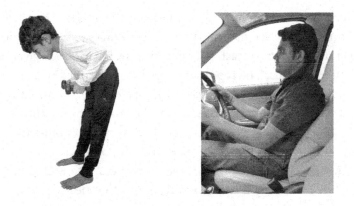

Rounded shoulders and hunched back postures at work show up during the day in daily activities like brushing teeth, eating, exercising and driving

An inefficient posture creates loss of mobility, which tightens tissues and creates imbalances even for fit individuals. The hours we spend on sedentary activities create body shapes that function with less efficiency. These inefficient shapes and postures that we are accustomed to being in all day will invariably get ingrained in us and are subconsciously carried forward to our daily functional movements like sitting, brushing teeth, driving and eating. Incorrect daily functional patterns create habits that further impact our movement and fitness activities. We condition the body to the shapes we use the most. An example of this can be seen in the hunched backs of a lot of the cyclists who very diligently cycle every morning on Marine Drive, Mumbai. The subconscious habit of a rounded back is ingrained in the body by hunching for long hours at work and this is completely counterproductive!

Being desk-bound for hours and having a passion for running can be biomechanically contradictory, as mobility is compromised right from the head to the ankles. That's why runners are seen limping after a marathon—we use our mind and willpower to reach the finishing line, but the body gives up after the race. The repeated stress of an unskilled movement pattern will eventually lead to injury or pain. Without any pre- and post-care, we carry these malfunctions into our lives, simply thinking that rest, recovery, physiotherapy or painkillers will take care of it. But the body can take only that much abuse and this capacity reduces with each passing year. Eventually it will give way, and with time, our ability to pursue our passions is lost.

Skill in our static and dynamic movements and postures through the day will help us move better before we attempt to move more.

Are We Investing in 'Health' or in 'Aids to Health'?

Everyone is doing their best to invest in health today. People ask me, 'What is the ideal chair to sit on? Which is the best one that money can buy? Which is the most comfortable one?' I say, 'Get the most uncomfortable one money can buy—it will give you the most comfort in the long run!'

The problems start when we get too comfortable and just don't want to move. Sitting is considered comfortable. *But sitting comfortably in a chair and experiencing no fatigue, pain and loss of mobility requires the art of efficient sitting, and that requires skill. There is no chair that can act as a substitute for efficient sitting.* People come in different shapes and sizes, so there cannot be a chair made for each individual that is just perfect. *If we understand the most optimal way to sit, we can use any chair, desk or gadget and use our intelligence to make it efficient and suitable to our purpose and our body's shape and size.*

Many are duped into buying ergonomic chairs, desks, pillows, computer mice, keyboards, posture braces and back supports but use them inefficiently. Consequently, they still suffer from the same aches and pains. How can anyone be motivated to use a standing desk if standing is disagreeable? *Ergonomically designed equipment is only beneficial for those who know how to sit, stand, position the body well and activate their muscles.* Changing your chair and adding a back support doesn't guarantee you will rid yourself of back pain. People think ergonomics is about choosing chairs and desks and adjusting a screen monitor, but that is just the tip of the ergonomic iceberg. There are no shortcuts to long-term health.

Today's world of sedentariness has made natural movement a back-breaking ordeal. Reconditioning and re-educating ourselves in the foundational movements— standing, sitting, walking, squatting, using our core etc.—is the first step before we get into ergonomics. *Learning how to optimally use furniture and gadgets needs to be combined with movement education.* This is the solution that this book offers and also the first step towards eradicating aches and pains from the body.

Money can buy the most expensive objects, like designer items. But does design have to compromise on comfort? I have visited people with the latest fancy furniture or designer pieces that decorate the corners of their homes. But I find myself playing musical chairs as on the one hand, design rarely comes with comfort. On the other hand, classical furniture that is comfortable can become very uncomfortable if you sink into the foam that hasn't been changed for a decade. When I see the homes of people who have substituted the regular sofa with a lounger to make it look more comfortable, I look in bewilderment at the little kids watching television with their lower back and stomach curved in, and I simply wonder how they will ever digest their popcorn? Since when has the illusion of comfort been able to delude us about what is truly enjoyable?

It is quite similar with a designer shoe. Does it come with the promise of retaining my natural mobility? Can I wear it comfortably for long hours without my feet hurting? The heels are slowly but surely changing the shape of my spine, and how I look in these shoes should not be more important than my feet lasting me a lifetime. *By definition, a luxurious shoe should make walking, standing and running feel easy!* But today, money buys arch supports and hard-soled shoes, which have become the new normal because our feet now need extra support! Since when has the use of external aids become normal and good for foot health?

Medicine today has advanced and provides solutions for the most injured or degenerated parts of the body. This is only for the lucky few who can afford it. But since when does an artificial knee or a stitched-up shoulder become a measure of good health?

With more money, I can opt to eat fresher, breathe fresher, move more in a natural environment so I can sleep like a baby and preserve the joints, bones and mental health I was gifted with. I can invest money in shoes that allow ease of movement. I can spend money on an education that balances the effects of modern use of technology and thus averts all lifestyle-related disease and illness. *The best investment is in 'health' itself and not in any 'aids to health'.*

Movement education is the most long-lasting health investment. External aids and supports are not the solution to eradicating aches and pains permanently. They can only help us if we know how to sit, stand and move efficiently while using them.

Addressing Movement Limitations before More Movement

Many ignore their existing dysfunctions and continue their fitness routines by altering their workouts and overall movements to avoid pain. Chandini, a mother of two children, 36 years of age, came to meet me. With sadness in her eyes, she murmured, 'I have to avoid squats and lunges, as my knee hurts. Even walking now has become painful. My workouts have become restricted to fewer movements, and I just can't lose weight.'

Restrictions in movement patterns can be worked on. Limiting the range and scope of overall movement just to avoid pain is moving against the law of nature.

Rohan, a marathon runner, 33 years of age, shared his concerns with me. He said, 'I have completely recovered from my back pain, but I still occasionally experience discomfort while bending and picking up things or while sitting and getting up in certain positions. I can't seem to push myself to increase my race pace, as my herniated discs bother me after a few kilometres.' The back pain might have allowed Rohan to complete his 21 km runs, but experiencing niggling issues throughout the day doesn't indicate qualitative movement health. After using the two-step method shared in this book, he was not only pain-free throughout the day, but he can now easily complete his runs in shorter periods of time, breaking his own records every year. Chandini managed to lose 20 kg effortlessly and continues to squat and lunge pain-free.

If you have knee pain, a typical yoga class will ask you to avoid certain poses, or the gym instructor will ask you to avoid squats and lunges. Some may think that age and degeneration come with a few handicaps, so it is acceptable if we can't sit on the floor or if we have other movement restrictions and limitations. *How many restrictions in our natural movements have been accepted and are unaccounted for in our lives because we have adapted to them? If we keep limiting our fundamental movements, we won't be able to condition the body to a wealth of overall activity, which enables us to function as normally as possible.*

Bending is bad for the back, squatting is bad for knees, the right way to lunge is when the knee isn't overshooting the ankle, sitting is bad—I have busted many of these myths in this book. Every individual even with the most complicated musculoskeletal issues, aches and pains can perform all these basic and inescapable movements all their life. Neeru, aged 64, had one knee surgically replaced. After a few years, she developed lower-back pain and was advised to replace the other knee. Today, she excitedly educates her friends and family on how simple changes in movement habits have altered her life in a substantial way. She neither needs the surgery nor the painkillers to ease the back pain.

Movement cannot *cause* discomfort and pain. It is the inept foundation of our untrained movements that are the predominant cause of pain.

Moving Efficiently with Skill Makes Movement Easy

Better movement and posture are by-products of efficient body mechanics.

The sign of mental success is when our nervous system is completely relaxed. That's when the best things are accomplished. Physical success is similar—it is determined when every movement and position is maintained with a sense of ease.

We might not know the correct technique when we observe an athlete engaged in a sport, but we recognize a good athlete from an average one just by the way they move. The good athlete will make what they do seem really easy. Like an adept dancer, a truly fit individual carries themselves with grace and proficiency in all movements throughout the day.

I won't avoid standing and choose to sit if I find standing comfortable. If I can lift heavy objects from the boot of the car or move a chair or table without my back giving way, then I am efficient. I won't avoid picking up heavy things if I am confident I will be able to lift them. Opting to squat, instead of bending, while I want to access something in the lower cabinets should feel natural. If I can climb two stairs in one stride, I won't hesitate to do so, since I'm proficient. If my neck and trunk can comfortably rotate to fetch something from the back seat of the car, or if I can twist to throw a Frisbee™ without feeling stiff, I am at ease because I have good mobility. If I am late and can run with my luggage to catch a flight, bus or train without huffing and puffing, then it is a measure of being physically fit, as everything happens with a 'sense of ease'.

How many of us recall saying, 'I don't want to do this movement because I don't like it!' You simply don't like it because you lack the *skill* to perform it. The same movement will be liked if it is 'easy'!

However, a movement that feels easy isn't always efficient. *The body adapts and gets better at withstanding any stress we expose it to, be it a poorly executed movement or a skilful one!* When the body adapts to easier patterns of movement and postures that may not be efficient or safe, it has the potential to harm us in the long run. For example, bending with a rounded back may seem easy, but it is very painful if you suffer from lower-back pain. Incorrect mechanics will eventually lead to loss of mobility, pain and setbacks—not an efficient, skilful one. Performing movement 'well' is the key, combining a focus on quality with the right quantity.

> We all expend energy in performing tasks and activities, but a skilled mover uses less energy as compared to an unskilled one.

Doing an activity with the least amount of energy is what makes movement easy. We are so enamoured by the outcome of reaching a certain weight goal or wanting to perform a bicep curl with a certain weight, or wanting to compete in a 50 km marathon, that we forget it is the *ease of the journey* that matters more than the goal itself! *Merely completing our target and feeling pain during or after the process takes away the satisfaction of accomplishing the goal.* 'Mind over matter' is necessary to complete a fitness goal, reach the finish line of a race or complete a certain quota of daily activity. But qualitative movement, coupled with a strong will, gives us a sense of satisfaction after achieving our goals because it is *injury-free.* Losing a leg while climbing Mount Everest was definitely not the aim! Suffering from tennis elbow as a result of attempting 30 kg bicep curls isn't really increasing strength. Inability to walk after completing a marathon isn't the mark of a winner. *Injury and pain imply a lack of skill and technique.* Weight loss should not feel like a chore that requires us to spend endless hours at the gym. Movement should be a natural and effortless part of our life—much like breathing. If moving is easy and natural, we need no motivation to move! We move because we enjoy it! *Less is more if we are skilled in movement.*

Not having qualitative movement patterns is the reason why many individuals can't and don't progressively increase their output in their physical activities for years on end. They will be walking the same number of kilometres or carrying the same weights, without their fitness really improving.

When we are talking about how to prevent setbacks in movement to enjoy continued and more movement, it is important to understand this: 'It's not the load that breaks us down, it's the way we carry it.'[2]—Lou Holtz, author of *Wins, Losses and Lessons.*

The right way to judge our efficiency in movement is to see if all the basic foundational movements—sitting, standing, walking, hinging, squatting, lunging, pulling, pushing, rotating, balancing and breathing—can be endured for long periods of time without any setbacks.

> Skill not only improves output and conserves large amounts of energy, but it also ensures safety and reduces risk of injury. An increase in output and strength will be a natural by-product of moving right.

Priming the Body before More Movement

Most individuals of all ages, including school-going children, have a sedentary life. Because of this, we need to first prime and prepare the body before undertaking any physical activity. For example, if I choose to go for my first hike or for one after a long time, I need to first prime and prepare the muscles that are used for hiking. My current choice of fitness activity might not give me the strength and mobility required for efficient hiking skills.

'I tried playing practice golf over the weekend just for a few hours, and my back started hurting,' exclaimed Vedika, 29 years of age. Many get dissuaded by pain and feel that a new sport or adventure isn't for them. 'I was playing racquetball every day for a month. Why have I suddenly developed a tennis elbow now?' says 26-year-old Pratik who has an IT job which requires him to sit at his desk all day.

Priming the body before trying out something new will increase your chances of success and will give you a natural boost to continue enhancing your physical fitness. If you haven't engaged in rotational movements in your life, then your back won't be prepared to handle the load of the golf club when you swing it. If you haven't ever used your wrist and forearm in sports or activities, your body will react to the sudden strain it experiences. This gap between preparation and execution needs to be filled by choosing more comprehensive movements in our regular fitness that address these goals. After understanding this scientifically, anaesthetist Dr Kavita, aged 55, enthused, 'In spite of standing all day in surgery, I have managed to renew my passion for Kathak. I move better today than I did in my thirties, as I complete intense routines with great ease and no pain or fatigue in the legs! I am sure I will continue to work and dance all my life!' Many walkers, runners and sports addicts share similar success stories, as the two-step programme featured in this book has been a life-changing methodology. Every individual, of any age and fitness level, can pursue their passions and effortlessly push themselves to achieve more by incorporating the two-step programme into their daily life.

What This Book Offers in a Nutshell

The COVID-19 work from home and home-schooling situation has increased sedentariness and musculoskeletal problems among both adults and children. Sitting on the floor or squatting, a basic functional movement, is on the decline, with an increase in the usage of a chair for everything. Any long-term sedentariness has its effects on our overall health and well-being. If we try to push ourselves to move more and be less sedentary, we may end up getting injured, and if we move less, we still face aches and pains and the perils of weight gain. Unfortunately, this is the complex web most of us are caught up in. So how do we escape from this trap and bounce back from a sabbatical of sedentariness? How can we increase movement safely without injury? Or to put it simply, how do we continue to reap the benefits of just feeling good and healthy, in any environment and at any time? How can we move easily, naturally, persistently and have fun at the same time? All these questions have their solution in these two steps:

Step 1: Relearning qualitative movement skills and posture for our daily life activities;

Step 2: Having a self-care programme that takes care of any repetitive stress on the body.

Most types of fitness and alternative treatments today fail to focus on the above aspects, leaving a busy individual with less time and resources to attend to these ignored areas of their health. Integrating these methods within our daily life as much as we can is essential and can take care of our specialized fitness needs while incorporating all the missing aspects. You will become a master at troubleshooting your own aches and pains instantly within minutes! You will save money and avoid endless trips to the doctors. The best part is that the self-care programme is easy to use in a home environment, in the office or while travelling, as it requires only minimal equipment.

How to Use This Book

All the technical knowledge used by specialists in their fields is shared in this book in an easy-to-understand guide that can be used practically. The two steps are a safe and life-changing solution for individuals of all ages, from children to the elderly, to use and benefit from. Paying attention to how we move and sit contributes largely to keeping our bodies pain-free. These simple changes in our daily-life movements, combined with the self-care programme, bring instant results for individuals facing pain. Even if you just want to improve your mobility and feel less stiff, the self-care programme works magic and the results are felt instantly!

Those who lack motivation to work on their health and put in that extra effort in a self-maintenance programme must know that even a few simple changes in daily life mentioned in this book can bring about transformations in health in unexpected ways! Small habits that we are mindful of, such as the way we hold our neck or the way we sit, can bring great ease to overall mobility in the body, which will protect us from current as well as future aches, pains and degeneration. These simple tips are meaningful additions to life, as they add to not only longevity but also better health for individuals of all ages.

Repetitive Stress in Static and Dynamic Positions

A single, inefficient position held statically for a prolonged period of time, or an unskilled movement of the body, both have the same amount of repetitive stress. Our skill in static as well as dynamic movements needs to be constantly improved, or else these movements will cause muscle, tissue or joint restriction and dysfunction over a period of time. *Static as well as dynamic postural quality is the first step towards a pain-free body.*

It is said that the 'best posture is always the next position'. Many think that taking a break after sitting every twenty minutes counters the damage caused to the body while sitting. The reason why emphasis is given to changing positions constantly is that if you stay too long in one position, the next position feels like an effort. That is how the human body functions. We should not get accustomed to any one position, as it works like 'emotional dependence' or our 'comfort zone'. For example, using a new phone with the latest technology is uncomfortable at first because we are used to the old one.

Check your position now. Are you too comfortable? Don't get too comfortable in any position, because the most comfortable position is also adding repetitive stress and is developing subconscious habits. This is why ideologies of 'moving more' were born. Changing positions frequently might be a good start for someone who sits for hours on end, but repetitive stress is much more complicated and requires more than just taking frequent breaks.

Through the day our backs are either in flexion or extension.

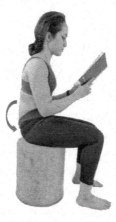

Flexion while relaxing, reading or during screen time

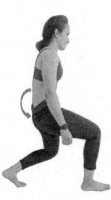

The same habit of flexion during exercise and daily movements

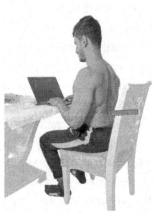

Extension during sedentary work hours or standing long hours

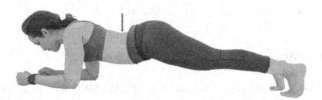

Extension during exercise and other daily movements
like bending or walking

We condition our brain with postural habits we repeatedly use most of the day. These same habits surface during the latter part of our day, such as during sleep. I have seen the poor bending habits or rounded backs in young children often infiltrate into their sleep. They are with their backs rounded even while they are asleep, as this posture held during the day feels comfortable at night.

In this golden age of physical fitness trends, the gap between true well-being and fitness continues to increase, as there are more injured individuals than fit ones. Most cannot align their spine to a plank because their brain doesn't know what a neutral spine position is while sitting, standing, bending or moving. These everyday flexion and extension faults are carried into exercise routines with compromised form. Even if emphasis is given on technique, the form is poor.

I urge adults and children to self-correct their movement habits at all hours of the day. This is for those individuals who are truly motivated to improve their health and well-being and want to keep moving competently at any age and benefit from their fitness programmes. This book details how to stand and walk better and reveals how pains can start with incorrect body mechanics and posture. Our feet are the foundation of the whole body and if we truly want to stay away from any medical condition, we need to reassess the way we distribute our body loads in all the positions we hold.

Summary

- My daily movements and my fitness choices should come with an assurance that they will prevent surgery, injury, aches and pains and degeneration.

- An indicator of good health and feeling good is how efficiently I can move over a sustained period of time—easily and free of aches and pains in all my daily-life movements as well as fitness routines. Even if our environment pushes us into sedentariness, I am in good health if I don't experience any aches and pains.
- Sedentary hours create inactive muscles and limit our mobility. Therefore, we must attend to these areas before we undertake a movement goal.
- External aids that claim to make us pain-free are merely band-aids and quick fixes. They are not solutions that eradicate aches and pains. They can only help us if we know how to sit, stand and move efficiently while using them. They may help for a short time, but the pain returns, as the original movement dysfunction in the body still exists. For example, individuals may wear arch supports, but their arches still collapse when they walk, despite wearing the support. External aids have to be combined with movement education, which is the most long-lasting and best health investment.
- Qualitative static and dynamic movements and postures are the first step towards staying pain-free. The second step is investing time in some self-maintenance to keep ourselves mobile. Skilled movement reduces mobility restrictions. Unskilled movements make the body tight and increases dysfunction. The more skilled we are at movement, the less time we need to spend on increasing and maintaining our mobility.
- An increase in output and strength is a natural outcome of moving right. We need not push through pain signals to move more.

- Avoiding the movements that cause us pain is not a solution. This limits our overall movement. Retraining our movements to perfect them is enough to stay pain-free.
- We must prime our body before getting into new movements to keep aches, pains and injuries at bay.

2

Posture

What Is Ideal Posture?

There is a lot of misinformation about what the 'ideal posture' of a body is.

Children are reprimanded when they slouch and asked to sit straight, but they simply correct this by overarching their lower back, which is even more detrimental to their posture.

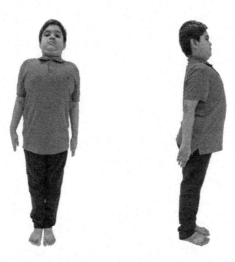

Over compensation is seen in the lower back
and the chest being thrust out excessively

There simply isn't enough education and awareness on what
the ideal spinal position is—the one that will cause the least
amount of degenerative changes. Most individuals who meet
me for the first time and know what I do, try to create a good
impression and thrust their chest out or stand with their
feet together, as they think that is good posture. But none
of these meet the standards of the 'ideal'. I once met a very
polished, sophisticated woman. She had the straightest back
and posture I have ever seen on an 80-year-old! She carried
herself with utmost poise, sitting and standing with her chest
held out, even at 80. Upon examining her, I discovered her
straight back to be intensely stiff! Unfortunately, all those
years of sitting perfectly erect had not served her well, as she
had lost out on spinal flexibility.

Flexibility classes today practise flexion and extension
poses that help in gaining spinal flexibility. But they do not

even touch upon the ideal of a neutral spine, which we need to maintain throughout the day.

Right Way to Bend Using the Hinge

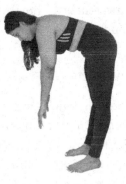 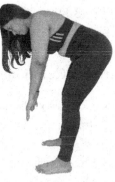

Bending forward incorrectly with a
straight back and hyper extended knees.

The correct way to bend
using the hinge.

Bending forward with a straight back without hinging is not a sign of qualitative movement, as it will create stress and strain on the knees and lower back and may cause degeneration.

Most people feel that posture can be corrected with simple measures such as thrusting their chest out. But this unenlightened perspective can be as hazardous as slouching. Incorrect posture has its effect as time passes, creating mobility restrictions as we subconsciously use these patterns through the day in everything we do.

Another hazardous belief many have is that one hour of exercise will counter the damage of twenty-three hours of bad movement and poor postural habits. Our fitness routines don't take into account the twenty-three hours of sloppy postures and shapes that our body has adopted. We move through life completely oblivious of the daily damage poor body mechanics cause, slowly but surely, even in children. There is a lot of misinformation about what it takes to be fit. Undue emphasis is given to strenuous routines targeted to achieving good looks with no awareness of how we are moving and carrying ourselves throughout the day.

Posture Is a Component of Movement

I have spoken a lot about posture, but what most understand about posture is that it is static. Posture is a part of movement— it is static as well as dynamic. Static posture is when we maintain one position, like sitting. Dynamic positions like walking also require qualitative movement postures. That way, each position we hold is a posture and has its own level of activity, depending on what we are doing. Individuals who don't exercise are known to have not only poor posture, but also poor movement mechanics. Due to a lack of body awareness, they maintain more static positions than dynamic ones. This is what differentiates a dancer from a cyber-person who maintains their seated position for most of the day.

The body was designed by nature to adapt intelligently to circumstances, just as everything else adapts in nature. Humans create dams, but water always finds a different path to flow in. It adapts. Similarly, our bodies adapt to develop into the shape of the position we use most. Our static postures can limit our dynamic ones. The functionality of the body depends on its flexibility, shape and comfort. The simplest definition of good posture is how comfortable and how much at ease we are in our own body. Posture is simply another word for position and varied positions are self-created movement patterns.

Good posture is often seen in elite athletes who are married to superior movement. Poor posture on the other hand, is seen in individuals who are completely oblivious to the major role that posture plays in physical health. A person may be born with knock-knees, bow-legs, scoliosis and kyphosis or may have a family history of bunions, but the symptoms only manifest and get aggravated with time because of inappropriate use of the body. Flawed usage of the body is an everyday choice we make—we can't excuse ourselves by saying, 'I can't help it, I have been like that since childhood.' *We are a certain shape because somewhere our poor postural positions have contributed towards creating it.*

Some people are so preoccupied that even if they experience pain because of a position that is causing postural stress, they are completely oblivious to it. They blame their lifestyle and the intense busy-ness of their day. 'My mind was obviously too busy and distracted to notice my posture!' 'By the end of the day, I got a catch!' *Awareness is generated only with repeated conditioning of good positions. That same intelligence then works on autopilot.* This requires time and patience and a self-maintenance programme.

An exaggerated awkward position like sitting crooked may feel uncomfortable instantly, within a few seconds or a few minutes, for people who have more vulnerable bodies. A younger, less vulnerable person may feel comfortable even in compromised positions. *But eventually, every exaggerated position will slowly create an imbalance in our tissues. Not experiencing any pain doesn't mean that there is no stress and strain on our tissue.*

Poor Posture, Postural Stress and Poor Postural Choices

These terms might sound similar, but they vary in application. These are all classic examples of *poor posture*:

- Sitting for hours with your legs crossed one on top of the other elevates the hip on one side (this leads to lower-back, hip and sciatica pain);[1] [2]
- Sitting on your wallet (leads to lower-back, hip and sciatica pain);[3]
- Working or eating with a hunched back (leads to respiratory and digestive issues);[4]
- Tucking your knees under a chair (makes knees stiff and may lead to knee pain);
- Sitting for long hours with legs crossed at the ankle (can change foot and shin structure);
- Standing with your weight only on one leg (changes the entire body's mechanics).

All these positions can be avoided through awareness, as there is a 'choice'. What can't be avoided is the *postural stress* caused by external environmental circumstances. These are unavoidable circumstances where we have no choice—for example, we may be forced to sleep while sitting in an aircraft, our job may force us to stand for long hours with no rest or breaks, wearing heels may be unavoidable,[5] or we may have a job, like that of a surgeon or chef, that requires us to constantly bend over for prolonged periods of time. A certain amount of stress is unavoidable in such circumstances. Many use external aids to ease the stress during that time, like a neck cushion while sleeping in the aircraft or wearing certain shoes that help you stand for long hours. These aids may ease the discomfort experienced, so most of us feel that they are a blessing. But in truth, nobody has made us aware of the underlying stress and strain that our tissues are still experiencing. The effect of postural stress surfaces when we go for a massage. Some body parts feel very tender and painful. This is why there is always a need for a periodic maintenance programme that flushes the stress out of our tissues. It helps restore and refresh our tissues so we don't reach the point of acute pain—the Move Better Mobility Course is one such programme.

Even the slightest tightness in the foot or back can cause movement deviations while bending or lifting something that we may not be aware of. Suddenly something will snap, and then it's just too late! *If our tissue quality is maintained, we can get away with some postural stress without facing major repercussions that may surface immediately or sometime later.*

Poor postural choices are the postures we willingly adopt because they are more comfortable, instead of being functionally optimal and balanced. An example is wearing a backpack only on one shoulder. Backpacks are built with two straps so that both can be used. We wear worn-out shoes just because we are too attached to how they feel. We choose a tight shoe or a closed-toed shoe just because it is the latest fashion. We sit on awfully designed furniture because of its aesthetic appeal or use mattresses and cushioned chairs and sofas in which the foam has worn out. We have the option of changing our mattresses every eight years but we don't, because it is too heavy on the pocket, but the postural stress we endure as a result of it is completely voluntary. We buy furniture and later realize it is uncomfortable. We can still hold on to it, but using it is a choice. Elevating the shoulder while talking on the phone because hands are too busy is also a choice.

After a while we realize that everything is always a choice, and there's always a better option if we choose to exercise it.

The Impact of Posture on Our Mental Health

Our body language is shaped by the sum total of our experiences. The way we move and our current body shape and posture is a reflection of our personality. Posture is the way we live and carry ourselves in the world. It reveals our stories, how we express ourselves and interact with our environment. It is a reflection of our everyday struggles and emotions. Posture can be used to understand human emotions. It can also be used to make judgements and create impressions in a social environment. Our posture mirrors our insides. It determines our success and stability even in mental and emotional wellness. We can understand our mental state and that of others better by analysing *open and closed postures*.[6]

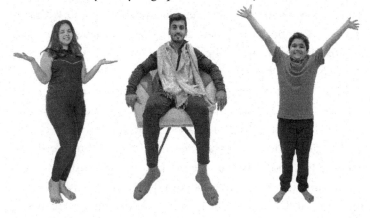

OPEN POSTURES

Open postures communicate to the observing individual that there is enough confidence, self-validation, warmth and openness of expression.

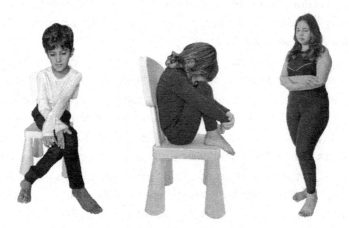

CLOSED POSTURES

Closed postures can give the impression of indifference, boredom, lack of confidence and introversion.

As we can see, the main distinction in closed and open postures is position of the hands. An easy way to become more positive and increase creativity is simply by rolling the arms out such that the palms face upwards. The arms set the position of the spine and prevent slouching.

Many people try to hide their emotions through sugar-coated words, but the body doesn't lie. Body language is not about what you say but how you say it. Research studies prove that non-verbal communication has a greater impact than verbal communication, as 65 per cent of the meaning we derive during interactions comes from non-verbal communication.[7]

Reading body language comes in handy for job interviews.[8] During an interview or when speaking in front of an audience, we all get only one chance to make a first impression. It is quite evident that success comes with good body language, and open postures play a significant role in this amongst other things.

Do you feel stuck in a certain thought or emotion? See what posture you are stuck in for most of the day! Happy movements and postures create happy, positive thoughts. Movement therapists bring about mental and emotional wellness to individuals who suffer from low self-esteem, illness, physical disabilities and emotional disturbances. If you are always in an open posture, your moods and self-esteem will typically be boosted, as energy levels are increased in the brain. Today, there is scientific data to back up this correlation between posture and moods. A San Francisco State University study[9] [10] observed how students' thinking changed when they were asked to recall negative and positive memories. They were asked to do this twice—once while in a slumped position and once while sitting upright. As much as 86 per cent of the students reported that it was much easier to recall negative memories in the slumped position, while 87 per cent found it easier to remember positive things while sitting in an erect position.

You are more likely to remember positive emotions connected to certain life experiences while walking upright.[11] Individuals who slouched often recorded negative emotions—bringing up the worst-case scenario in their experiences. The conclusion of these studies is that altering body posture to a more upright position can elevate mood and energy levels.

Dr Erik Peper of San Francisco State University has also conducted studies that indicate children with good posture score better at math tests. Other studies correlate learning outcomes with posture as well. They claim closed postures have a negative impact on mental processes, which affects cognitive skills, while open postures do exactly the opposite.

Dr Peper's research also reveals that musicians and athletes who have good posture have better performances. There is a decrease in energy and increase in helplessness, hopelessness, powerlessness and self-defeating thoughts when the person habitually looks down in a slouched position.[12] Other researchers have found that office workers are more prone to anxiety and depression than manufacturing workers.[13] This, they say, could be attributed to the hours of sitting and slouching at a desk.

Posture affects our emotions, and emotions also affect our posture. In the book *Bioenergetics*, Alexander Lowen explains, 'a jaw which is held by tense muscles may hold back impulses to bite. A tightly contracted throat inhibits the expression of crying or screaming but the person may not be conscious of this inhibition until he tries to cry or scream. Rigid shoulders may block impulses to strike out in anger.'[14] The deep psychological connection between the emotions the mind experiences can make muscles contract, which leads to tension blocks. Over time these contracted muscles with trapped emotions affect our posture and the way we move.

When we experience negative emotions, stress, anxiety and depression, they influence the formation of muscles and alter the body's appearance and structure. Many want to change the way they feel without trying to analyse their emotions or incurring the costs of counselling. Changing our posture is an easier first step to start feeling good. This is not to suggest that it is a substitute for therapy, but simply an add-on that makes you feel better instantly.

Even sleeping posture can affect one's mental health. People who sleep on their backs may experience a block in their nasal passages. The body has its own intelligence and uses the mouth to breathe instead of the nose. It's a well-known fact that mouth breathing increases thirst, clogs up the sinuses, increases the risk of sleep apnoea (1 million cases in India every year)[15] and disrupts sleep. Clogged sinuses and poor quality of sleep affect concentration and reduce mental output.[16]

Should I Take My Posture and Movement Health Seriously?

A closed posture is not always harmful. When facing danger, the body feels fear and uses a closed posture. It is a natural, automatic reflex for self-protection.

But prolonged use of a closed posture is a sign to the body of continual fear and stress, even when there is no imminent danger! Stress and anxiety affect 74–88 per cent of the Indian population, adopting open postures is a signal to the brain to de-stress, be optimistic and feel a sense of safety, peace and joy.

Often, we see Indian women slouching to conceal their breasts because they are very conscious of them. This is a protective response, which reflects insecurity and fear of social stigma. Women feel second best. *Now, imagine spending years in this position, which is constantly signalling to the brain to adopt a submissive attitude. This has a deep impact on moulding the personalities of women from early childhood.*

I encourage women to hold themselves in a better posture, keeping in mind their preferences by wearing scarves or stoles. This has a tremendous psychological benefit, with added improvement in breathing functions. *Movement expertise improves psychological health by creating a sense of self-efficacy and boosting self-esteem—the ingredients of success.*

We live in a world of start-ups, where there is a need for creative ideas and constant innovation. Some of the best ideas come when the body and mind are charged. We have heard the James Redfield quote, 'Where attention goes, energy flows.' When I roll my shoulders back with the palms facing outward, it is a sign to the universe that I am open and I welcome all good things. These come only to those who are open and receptive. A confident, lively, active and open person will assume the expansive position. The benefits are relaxation, joy and clarity. You don't feel stressed, listless, helpless or lethargic but instead cheerful, lively and dynamic. How are you sitting right now? With your arms folded across your chest? Is your body stooped? *Posture affects the way we learn and process information. The transmission of signals that come from the brain isn't optimal when the spine isn't aligned.* So uncross those legs and arms and be the architect of your own future.

3

Relearning Our Foundational Movement Principles

My years of study led me to an interesting observation. *The causal link between musculoskeletal issues and the repetitive stress caused by our job, hobby, routine activity and lifestyle is the underlying factor responsible for the misery of ill health.*

Our daily movements, in our occupation and hobbies, play a major role in exposing the body to repeated stress. Without this understanding, a person gets trapped into a cycle of self-sabotage.

I met 24-year-old Rajlata, a vivacious girl, working in a law firm. She woke up every morning with a headache that lasted through the day. On questioning, she said, 'I work 12 hours a day on the computer, and in the evening I go to a boxing class for fitness.' Aa-ha! Slouching in a chair for long hours, followed by an intense punching session. Tight chest muscles precipitated by slouching is the perfect recipe for neck strain and a concomitant headache. Even a young girl cannot escape these consequences!

Examples of repeated stress on the lower back are seen in the occupation of surgeons, who bend over for hours daily during a surgery. Nurses and dentists experience the same stress during their workday. Imagine a dentist, who already has the repetitive stress of bending all day at work, going home to attend to his/her newborn baby. Without any sort of maintenance programme to keep that back strong to last a lifetime, they are definitely going down the path of self-created misery. Dentists have a higher risk of developing lumbar herniated intervertebral disc (HIVD) due to prolonged sitting and improper postures during work.[1][2] Back and neck pains are inevitable for homemakers with poor bending and slouching habits while they attend to their children all day or use gadgets inappropriately. Among the youth, the pain in the elbow caused by taking multiple selfies is known as the 'selfie elbow'. Many must have experienced pain in the thumb due to the 'texting thumb'. The efficient way to type on a phone without stressing the thumb is quite simple—use the index finger.

Let's see some occupations that have repetitive stress on the neck—a chef, diamond sorter or pathologist who has to constantly look down every day. To this, if they add a game of chess, playing cards or reading as a hobby, it becomes the perfect equation for permanent neck pain. Holding the neck in an efficient position, coupled with a maintenance programme, is required to rid themselves of the dowager's hump, which protrudes behind the neck. An incorrect forward head posture can lead to blocked ears, migraines, jaw pain and tension headaches. People using the mobility programme shared in this book are aghast when they discover how tight their jaw is and are surprised with the connection between their headaches and jaw tightness.

When the body is active in one position for a prolonged period, it gets accustomed to staying that way. Thus, we create shapes such as rounded shoulders, hunched backs, crooked spines, collapsed arches and duck feet in our body. Most individuals who have rounded shoulders and forward head postures are shallow breathers, with reduced lung function. Some may even experience breathlessness occasionally because the chest becomes tight! Young boys and girls run to take ECGs or stress tests and are completely perplexed when they are released with an all clear. But the reasons for their chest pain remains a mystery. Breathlessness, tightness in the chest, acid reflux—these are all symptoms of the repetitive stress on our tissue due to poor postural and movement habits. The forward head posture that continues to degenerate over the years makes basic functions like swallowing also difficult.

Many people are also unaware that their chronic acid reflux, causing heartburn, is intrinsically linked to their posture. According to Dr Kyle Staller of Harvard Medical School, heartburn and slow digestion are caused by 'slouching as it puts pressure on the abdomen which forces stomach acids to flow in the wrong direction'.[3] If you are one of those who experience digestive issues, check to see if you are slouching while eating or after eating. We may find our postural habits and everyday simple movement patterns very trivial and insignificant, but most injuries, aches, pains and ailments don't just occur by chance or because of age—they are the result of long-term abuse of body parts.

Different occupations make different demands and put different stresses on the body. An accountant, architect, cashier or lawyer working all day at the computer is prone to developing rounded shoulders and thoracic tightness.

Sonographers regularly working on an ultrasound machine will commonly experience fatigue and pain in the neck and shoulder due to repetitive stress on the arm holding the machine. Many photographers have come to me complaining that their shoulder, elbow and neck hurts from holding heavy cameras for prolonged hours. Have you ever experienced this if your hobby is photography? Even women carrying heavy designer bags on their arms can suffer from pain in the elbow and shoulders.

Frequent air or road travellers as well as pilots develop back and hip problems, which result from continuous sitting and sleeping on poorly designed chairs, cars and aeroplane seats. Many sit with one leg crossed over the other, which tilts the hip and deforms the lower back.

Some professions require individuals to stand for long hours, as with salespersons and hospitality personnel, teachers, doctors, etc. They have an advantage over seated occupations as they get to burn more calories standing and walking. But if they inefficiently distribute their body load, they are prone to inflammation, varicose veins, foot pain and other complications of the feet. Improper foot positions like fallen ankles and arches affect the knees and lower back in the long run. Many of us, while standing and waiting in queues, are likely to stand with more weight on one leg and may even have the hip jutting out. This postural laziness, which many don't consider a big deal, has the capacity to wreck the spine in later years. Habits become shapes, and shapes have consequences, as unequal loads will eventually wear out our joints.

Foot problems are common among most individuals, for example; Achilles tendinitis, plantar fasciitis, bunions affect around a million Indians a year.[4] Improper foot mechanics later change the shape of our bones; thus, we see many with bow legs and knock knees that require knee surgery.

People are aware if they have flat feet or not. Yet, even when they don't have flat feet, many are talked into buying footwear with arch supports! Ignorance makes the gullible individual think they are doing everything in their hands to improve their foot health and pain by buying external aids and supports. The industry that markets aids for flat feet has become very fashionable and offers them as a shortcut to magically correct improper flat feet and get rid of pain. But for most individuals, the pain comes back in a different form after a few years, not necessarily in the foot, but in the knee or lower back, and they don't make the connection between the two. For the majority who use arch supports, postural laziness only increases with time. The corrective measures taken don't remove the stress on the joints completely, as the overall gait is still faulty. When the root of faulty mechanics is not addressed by a return to natural poise, the external aids will not give permanent relief. I have met the unlucky few who have used all possible external aids, but still have had to go down the road of opting for knee replacements and lower-back surgery. That is why it is crucial to bring back awareness to the foundational principles of movement, elaborated below. Users can differentiate between the real common-sense approaches to realign our body, vis-à-vis new-age smart fixes.

When Deepa from Bengaluru, 28 years old, came to me, she said she used to take up a new fitness class every year, which was great fun in the beginning, but despite all the time and money invested, she never felt like she was progressing in her fitness. Every time she attempted any form of fitness activity, aches and pains in different areas of the body would surface. After she improved her basic movement skills, she developed all-round fitness in strength, flexibility and breathing skills.

A sudden boom in fitness fads all over social media is great for seeking motivation, but the reality is that the quality of our musculoskeletal health hasn't improved. Not everyone is interested in longevity, as old age brings a loss of cognition that makes living that much more difficult. But everyone wants to live a pain-free healthy life that is qualitative, however long that may be. *We need to retrain ourselves in the basics of movement before we get into complicated exercises that the fitness world throws at us as bait, with all their starry-eyed promises. Our skill in all the foundational movements contributes towards actualizing those goals.*

The quality with which we perform our foundational movements has a direct impact on the efficiency of the more advanced compound movements in exercises. I know so many young people who avoid dead-lifts despite having personal trainers because they experience pain. The technique of dead-lifting can magically become a natural skill that can be polished with training and practice for a person of any age, who has perfected the basic skill of a hinging movement. The foolish will keep this basic movement at bay and miss out on the functional strength gained and the chance of developing a stronger back.

Besides exercise, the foundational movements seep into all aspects of our daily life. If I avoid some foundational movements, there is a lapse in my functional movement patterns, and this will affect other movements. Just like pathology gets complicated over time—where one medication for a disease has its side-effects and creates a chain reaction of other problems needing other treatments—it is a similar case with our movement mechanics. Faulty movements and avoidance of certain movement patterns create many deviations in our overall mechanics. Thus, one issue leads to another in succession. When we get injured, we may blame the exercise, sport or the situation we were in. But after implementing the right way to move better, we realize that there were many lapses in our basic movements that led to the injury. Improving our foundational movement skills is necessary so that we don't complain about the level of difficulty of exercises or feel that movements or daily-life chores are too strenuous. When we don't pay heed to the foundation, we inevitably go back to the same erroneous movements, with the same aches and pains as consequences. Paying attention to merely treating pain symptoms is like rinsing clothes without removing the dirt!

In some parts of the world where ancient culture, work habits and living habits have been preserved, people stay fit and move well even in their 90s. Enhancing our movement mechanics allows us to attain levels of optimum health and wellness and stay youthful through our entire lifespan.

The foundational elements of movement are as follows: spinal stabilization, breathing, standing, walking, hinging, squatting, lunging, balancing, pulling and pushing and rotational stability and strength. The standard 'ideal' every individual should aspire to is described below.

Standing Better

First stand well before you walk, then walk well before you run.

Standing is the foundation of movement. If we don't stand well, we won't move well either. Individuals who stand for long hours get tired, feel pain and sometimes don't recover from the previous day's stress easily. Elevating the legs every day for twenty minutes can give relief,[5] but a better foundation reduces stress and fatigue and decreases the time spent on recovery.

Neutral Standing Posture

The Feet

The foundation of standing well starts with the feet. If you have wide hips and small feet or narrow feet, it is likely that you will face unequal loading patterns. This also applies to individuals with smaller heels as compared to the forefoot. These examples of different foot structures are not an impediment to movement or reason enough to cause pain, if we are mindful of how we distribute our body weight efficiently on the feet, irrespective of the structure we are born with.

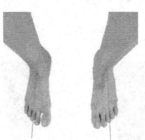

Keeping the feet straight
Keeping the toes pointing straight ensures equal foot pressure

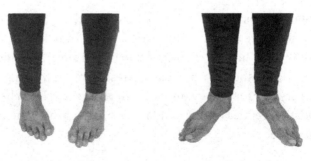

Pigeon toed feet   Duck shaped feet

We may have never thought that a simple thing like keeping our toes pointed straight while standing is important. Pigeon toes/in-toeing or having duck feet/out-toeing leads to unequal loading patterns that lead to incorrect gait. The shape of the foot can alter the entire structure of the body including the knees, hips and lower back.

A neutral foot position has the toes separated wide apart, pointing forward. This distributes the load of our body equally on all mounds of the base of the foot. It also ensures a wider foundation that can carry body weight efficiently. This method of standing reduces fatigue and foot pain and makes standing and walking enjoyable.

Keeping a neutral arch

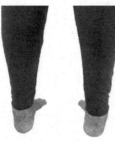
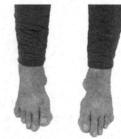

Supinated feet

Constant pressure on the outsides of the feet is called supination. This creates uneven loads and, in some cases, it can change the alignment of the knee and ankle.

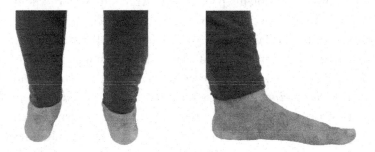

A pronated foot has a dropped arch or no arch

When the arch of the foot collapses inward (fallen arches) it is called over-pronation. You will know you have an over-pronated foot if you come across these five indicators—duck feet, collapsed arches, valgus knees, a curved Achilles tendon and lopsided worn-out shoes.

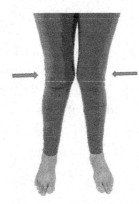

Knock-knees/valgus knee

An over-pronated foot leads to many problems with the knees, hips and lower back. Painful soles, feet and ankles, bunions, shin splints and Achilles tendon pain are some of the common problems people face. Arch supports or shoes having inbuilt arch supports are usually considered the solution to the fallen arch or flat-feet problems and have become big businesses. But this is a provisional bandage. Rarely do individuals have complete flat feet. *The arches only collapse due to the way the ankle is habituated to drop.* So, those who have become accustomed to using arch supports but don't have flat feet should check if the fault lies in the ankles instead of the arch. Learning to raise the arch naturally and reposition the ankle well is the natural long-term solution to better movement mechanics. *You cannot replace good foot mechanics with external aids and expect long-term pain-free outcomes.*

Many individuals report becoming pain-free after using arch supports, but after a few years, the pain returns in different parts of the foot, since the body loads have been displaced. Changing our foot mechanics to load them naturally, correctly and efficiently prevents the need for knee replacements and reduces lower disc degeneration. *External aids merely delay the onset of degeneration.* The after-effects may leave you with no option but surgery. Regularly mobilizing the ankles and a routine that incorporates foot releases restores the natural foot function.

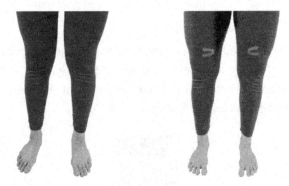

Generating a natural neutral arch is simple:

- Keep the feet always stacked under the hip. Always align your hip joint to the knee and ankle.
- Keep the toes pointing straight.
- Create a force towards the outer side of the foot but still ground the big toe. This ensures the weight is on the entire sole of the foot.
- Roll the inner thigh outwards to align the knee with the ankle. Another advantage of this technique is that it ensures that the knees are not hyperextended and are relaxed for individuals who stand with knees locked. With this, the knee cap isn't jammed in, and there is a natural lift in the arch.
- Separating the toes is difficult for those who have squashed toes and lack space in between. Wearing toe separators can help with this issue.

How to Stand Better

1. While keeping the feet pointed straight, try to spread out the toes. By separating the toes regularly, you will find that the sole of the foot becomes less tight and less painful during releases or massages.

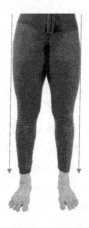

2. Many individuals stand with their feet close to each other. This creates more pressure on one leg than the other. For equal distribution of load, it is always better to stand with the legs hip-width apart. This aligns the pelvis, knee and ankles right under each other so that our bones stack perfectly one on top of the other. Sometimes I even encourage individuals who stand a lot to take a broader stance while standing, just for a change in position. This helps reduce fatigue.

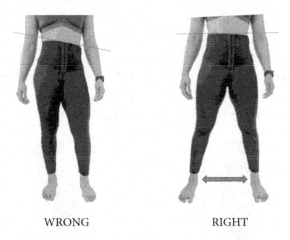

WRONG   RIGHT

3. Roll the inner thighs out to align the knees with the ankles.
    (refer to the figures above) This ensures the knees are not
    hyperextended or excessively bent and are relaxed. There
    is a natural lift in the arch.

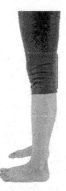
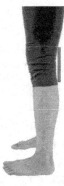

Hyperextended knee   A soft knee that is not
that jams and locks the knee   hyperextended nor excessively bent

4. Make sure the pelvis is not thrust forward causing sway back or an anterior tilt. To avoid these compensations, brace the midsection by 20 per cent and squeeze the glutes 50 per cent. This sets the lower back in place and stabilizes the trunk. An anterior–posterior balance is created, and the body naturally finds its centre of gravity.

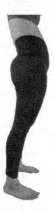 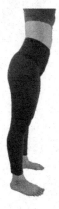

Sway back posture   Anterior tilt

5. As children, we might recall elders asking us to sit straight. Typically, we misinterpreted this by thrusting the ribcage forward and sticking out the chest. This isn't a neutral position for the upper trunk, as it tightens the spinal muscles. The ribcage should be tucked in and the shoulder blades rolled back and pushed down. This facilitates better diaphragmatic breathing. A mark of rounded shoulders is the position of the palms. If the palms face forward, then you qualify for rounded shoulders. This can simply be corrected by rotating the palms to face sideways.

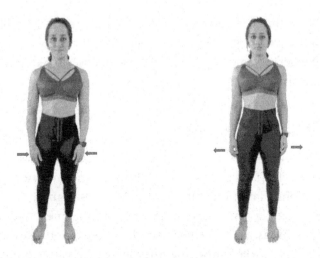

This naturally sets the shoulder blades in position without adjusting the shoulder or shoulder blade or moving the chest. Many people constantly roll the shoulders back. While it may feel good for some, it unnecessarily tightens the upper trapezius muscles, which are already overactive and tight. *Setting the shoulder in position is more about setting the shoulder blade rather than the actual shoulder.*

6. Lastly, keep that chin tucked in. It may look like you have a double chin, but it ensures you don't stick your neck out. The ideal position of the neck clears the passage for optimal nasal breathing, which is naturally deep and slow. It also prevents the neck from getting tight.

Walking Well Before We Run

Dynamic individuals as well as paraplegics value freedom of activity and always find ways of adding joy and fulfilment to life with more movement. Some of the fondest memories people have are of group hikes and long walks as they climbed hills together, enjoying the challenges and breathtaking views on the way.

Walking Meetings

Movement of the body is the representation of work in action. This is why some great thinkers and inventors like Steve Jobs, Harry Truman, Charles Dickens, Sigmund Freud and Aristotle have known to walk during meetings and consultations, as this helped them find inspiration.[6] Research on walking meets shows that they increase creative thinking even up to 60 per cent by some estimates.[7] Creative thinking[8] usually results in more productive meetings. A change in setting can provide inspiration, more flexible thinking and better problem-solving abilities. You will look forward to your day, as you may perceive it as fun! Even simply choosing to stand or walk while you communicate with employees or co-workers can generate a multitude of ideas and bring about stimulated communication. The energy levels after a walking meeting can shoot up, leaving you feeling lively and energized. This will improve efficacy at work even after the walking meeting has ended.

Walking Well

Walking is a biological process that is self-taught. But, as stated earlier, a lack of awareness and mobility maintenance can lead to inefficient gait patterns. Below is a list of a few of the common abnormalities while walking that are usually not thought of as problems that need attention. Try to identify them or ask a friend to see if you have any of these symptoms.

- Does your *hip drop* or sway side to side? It can be a sign of gluteal muscle weakness, called the trendelenburg gait.[9]
- Do you have a slight *limp*? Favouring one leg while bearing weight indicates that there may be a joint dysfunction.
- Do you *drag* your feet? This occurs if the heels don't lift off the ground through the full range of motion.
- Do you walk like a *duck*, with feet turned out? It will eventually wear out the knees and tighten the hip.

Our movement efficiency right after we get out of bed determines how much and how far we can move effortlessly until the last few steps at the end of the day. You can easily compromise on the quality of movement, especially if you are trying to complete your whole quota of physical activity of the day in the last two hours of the evening because your pedometer shows you a mere 4000 steps! An active lifestyle has great benefits and is essential, but even active and healthy individuals can suffer from aches and pains that may surface while trying to push the limit in order to meet a set target or to complete their goals in less time. Qualitative gait patterns can help a walker push through that extra kilometre effortlessly. The repetitive stress of poor gait patterns and no maintenance eventually leads to tightness in areas of the feet, calf and shin. Ankle sprains, knee pain, lower- and mid-back pain, foot pain and cramps that freeze the muscles are some other symptoms that appear in our lower extremities. These impediments lead to breaks in consistency of activity, eventually limiting our potential to advance further. *Moving well is all about effective time management. Once you start moving better, the need for maintenance reduces, saving valuable time and added effort.* The deviations from the ideal standing posture are reflected in our walking. *We may think that a few aches and pains are natural and they are a part of life. However, if you find these irritants affecting your mood and desire to move and perform, remember that you have a way out. It all boils down to how much time you wish to invest in staying pain-free and moving efficiently.*

Once you have mastered the correct standing position, walking should be the next in line. The steps listed below are the principal measures that need to be mastered well for an ideal gait.

- Keep the feet straight and toes pointed forward while you walk.
- The feet should always be hip-width apart when we walk and not too close to the centre of the body.
- Engage your core by 30 per cent, as it holds your trunk and prevents slouching.
- As you place one foot forward, squeeze the buttock of the back leg that is extended. This is essential as you don't want to overuse your hip flexors, especially during uphill climbs. The glutes are the largest muscles of the body and have more endurance.
- Landings should be gentle on the heel or mid-foot, as it is a sign of agility. No heel striking.
- If the foot is stiff, it will not allow a good take-off. Ensure there is enough mobility in the sole of the foot so that the arch lifts with each step.
- Take smaller steps so you don't over stride. This will prevent excess load on the calf muscle, making it less tight.

It will also propel you to walk faster. Think of babies and how their tiny steps make them brisk walkers. Remember, it is not distance but the calories and steps that matter.

First walk, then run, then practise walking and running on different terrains. If we see the example of good athletes, like cricketers or tennis players, we see that they can perform the same movements on various terrains. Cricketers bowl on different pitches and tennis players adapt to playing on grass and clay. Running on a track versus running on roads, versus running on rugged, rocky terrain can all present a different challenge to the breath and body. This is why there is a great need for us to match our fitness to the various hobbies and goals we want to attain. If I am preparing for a marathon or a hike at a specific altitude and terrain, then my fitness needs to match that. Lastly, remember to stop when you're walking badly. Overdoing with bad form is a prescription for pain and distress. There is always a tomorrow to get better in every way. Moving better comes first, then maintenance and then moving more. This is how we attain our fitness goals.

How to Find the Right Shoes

Primitive humans always walked and ran barefoot or used minimalistic footwear. Shoes were originally invented to protect the feet from getting bruised. They started off as being minimalistic to becoming fancier through the centuries. Fancy shoes that interfere with the way our foot lands and takes off, alter our natural gait pattern thus creating unequal body weight on our feet. This leads to degenerative changes in our foot structure over time. Cushioned shoes and shoes with built in arch supports are looked upon as a solution for preventing pain and injury. That is a flawed perception. Changes in foot structure can occur due to various types of shoes.

Hard-soled Shoes

By nature, the foot is designed to be flexible, as it bends and lifts naturally while walking. If we are accustomed to wearing only hard-soled shoes, the flexibility of the foot base and arch gets affected. They also prevent the ankles from naturally stabilizing the foot, and thus they become restricted and jammed. Stiff ankles further alter your gait, as you need to swing the foot around as you can't bend it to land on the next step.

> Keeping the soles of our feet supple should be a priority while choosing footwear.

Pointed, Tight Shoes

Shoes that squash the toes create dysfunction in the entire body. When our base is not anchored, imbalance is created in foot pressure. Thus the body manoeuvres itself into handling load and adapts, but this impacts our lower back and knees. Shoes that are raised in the front elevate the toes and cause unnecessary hyper-extension. Just as our bodies don't do well in one position, keeping the toes and feet in an unusually awkward position for too long is risky. Pushing the feet into tight shoes that compress the toes may look fashionable, but this increases the risk of bunions and valgus knees.

If we observe our feet, the forefoot and toes are usually broader than the heel. This shows how much body weight our forefeet are capable of handling. Many of the joints in the toes get stiff, and even if we are working towards maintaining mobility in them, pushing them into a squashed, crowded shoe becomes counterproductive!

> A broad toe-box should be a priority while choosing footwear.

High Heels

Any footwear that raises the heel above floor level is a heel. It can be a one-inch heel used by men or a five-inch one used by women! Anything that is not ground level, zero drop, doesn't resemble your natural barefoot stance is a heel worth discarding, or let's say, using sparingly. Heels are responsible for a change in the way our body handles load. The body is designed to adapt and adjust to gravity, so in order to balance, it will compensate elsewhere.

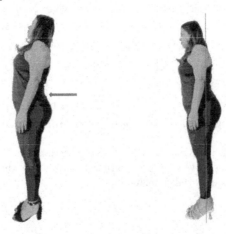

In the first picture above, we can see that wearing heels can result in excessive arching of the lower back which can in turn lead to back pain if the heels are worn for a long duration.

In the second picture, we can see that wearing heels can also make the body lean forward to compensate.

These are the ways in which the body's natural tendency to restore balance gets altered. We can also see how a heel can change the alignment of our entire body's structure! The higher the heel, the more the body tips forward. The body compensates in other ways, such as excessively arching the lower back or pushing the pelvis forward, creating a sway back posture. Knees can become permanently bent for those who regularly wear heels, with lower-back pain[10] being the most common symptom experienced. Heels create tightness in the muscles of the posterior chain. To counteract the harmful after-effect of these compensations of the body and the unnatural positions the body adopts as a result, some maintenance needs to be done. Many women with hyper-mobile joints* usually trip or sprain their ankles periodically, because wearing high heels increases hypermobility in the ankle.

Some individuals have an excessive heel strike. Heel striking is when we can hear a person's footsteps as they walk, which gets louder when they run. Excessive heel strike can be the cause of a lot of aches and pains for regular walkers and runners. Cushioned shoes and wearing heels shorten your heel cord, which creates excessive heel strike as the ankles get stiff. Landing on the mid-foot while running is considered the

---

* Hyper mobile joints are joints that are very supple and have an unusually large range of movement. This occurs in individuals when the tissues holding the joint together are too loose.

most 'neutral' strike, as it is low impact. So if you can hear the sound of your heel while walking, you know your heel strike is excessive.

> Choosing a shoe with a zero-heel drop that mimics a barefoot stance is a priority while choosing the right shoe.

Slippers/Flip-flops

Flip flops or slippers may seem like a minimalistic choice of footwear, since they are flat, but they come with their own limitations. They make the sole of the foot tight and lead to hammer toes,[11] since you need to clench the toes to prevent the slipper from sliding off the foot. Lifting the big toes automatically raises the arch of the foot. Clenching the toes is simply the opposite—it leads to tightness in the plantar fascia.

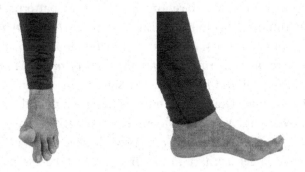

Lifting the toes is also a simple exercise people with flat feet must regularly do in order to keep the muscles of the arch alive. *Being barefoot naturally trains the abductor hallucis muscle. So those who walk barefoot most of the time naturally*

have better developed arches. Think before you wear those flip-flops at home. Your feet are missing out on an opportunity to naturally develop those arches!

Get rid of those house slippers and walk barefoot at home as much as possible.

Choosing the Right Footwear

Regular use of footwear that doesn't match the foot's natural ability to move will alter its patterns. A zero-drop (with no heel), flexible soft-sole shoe that doesn't elevate the toes or squash them is the key when hunting for shoes. I recommend wearing floaters with or without toe separators for walks, if they meet all the above criteria. Getting a shoe that doesn't meddle with our natural foot structure is the safest and surest way to retaining natural gait patterns, long-term joint health and becoming pain-free.[12] *But wearing the right shoes isn't a substitute for regular maintenance. The shoes are merely protection for the soles of the feet and not a solution for the repetitive stress that our tissues endure while moving.* The human body is designed to endure a lot of movement. We can push ourselves to walk kilometres on end as well as run at any age, provided we maintain what we have to get us there in the first place—the feet and legs. Soft-tissue release can accomplish this. You should not start a run or walk with a nagging discomfort from the previous day. The right approach would be to fix it so you can perform better than yesterday. *Unmanaged pain and injury eventually cost more money, and enduring pain requires that much more mental strength. You either spend time on prevention, or money on cures!*

Counterproductive Use of Foot Supports

We have already seen that many of the problems of the back, hip and knee start with the feet. There is no scientific evidence or research that proves cushioned shoes and arch supports provide better balance and alignment and a reduction in injuries, plantar fasciitis and knee pain.[13] External aids for the feet are used today as a quick fix for pain relief from an abnormality that was created progressively with poor use of the feet. If you have flat arches and valgus knees, your muscles are tight and the sole as well as your heel cords are stiff—no external equipment will fix these! A quick fix may give relief from pain, but eventually, it may alter gait patterns yet in another way.

Beena, 68 years old, flew down from Jaipur to meet me. She had been using arch supports for her flat feet for the last ten years. Her original pain in the ankles simply shifted to the top of the foot as years progressed. So the arch supports were not a permanent solution. Restoring Beena's foot, ankle mobility and retraining her gait so that it resembled her natural barefoot walking, helped her get rid of her pain. Even if we invest in shoes with a ready-made arch support, every human foot by nature is designed uniquely, and one size doesn't fit all. People who unnecessarily wear arch support shoes, thinking they are healthy and a wise choice, can supinate the foot while walking and running. With time, they develop stress fractures and inflammation on the opposite side of the foot. The ready-made arch supports and the arch support shoes come with a certain height and cannot cater to our personal foot design. Thus, despite using an arch support, the arch still collapses for some individuals. The safest and most efficient way out is to load the feet naturally by using our own body right. Many individuals have become pain-free by restoring their natural gait simply by regularly mobilizing and strengthening the foot muscles, and several have postponed knee surgery indefinitely, as the body begins to handle load better without pain. Initially one fears throwing away the external supports, but walking barefoot feels like a baby taking its natural first steps. Can you remember the last time when there were no aches and pains in your body? *Nature eventually restores balance, so it is better to gradually transition from using external supports and shoes to becoming more dependent on our natural internal support that we were born with—our feet.*

Productive External Aid

If you are a lover of external aids, you can use one of my favourite one: the toe separator. Scientific research proves that regular use of it actually works in reduction of valgus toes/ bunions, when combined with a maintenance programme of regular mobilizing.[14] It spreads the toes apart to create a larger base for the foot and keeps the sole of the foot from getting tight. Elderly people report regaining sensation and mobility in their stiff toes after regular use of these, just for a few hours a day. But remember, external tools work only when used alongside maintenance exercises. The foot has thirty-three joints, twenty-six different bones and over a hundred muscles, tendons and ligaments, so one solution can't be the magic wand to meet all the needs of the feet.

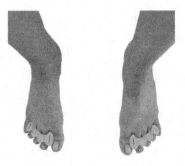

Stabilizing the Spine Better—the Core

Abdominals are a hot topic of discussion today. Every other person, from an executive to an 80-year-old, wants a flat tummy. When we think of the abdominals, we think of crunches and sit-ups, assuming they will burn belly fat. Sorry to burst the bubble—they don't! You may try out various fitness platforms that sell big numbers, but they do not necessarily deliver better movement or functional capability. I met Monica, 79 years of age, who was troubled with incontinence. 'It gets very embarrassing in social gatherings and long journeys, where one cannot find a washroom. It is also a problem whenever I cough, as when I cough I leak!' Once she started learning to strengthen her core, not only did her leaking bladder improve, but the hump in her back also straightened out. Even at 80 years of age, we can improve our internal functions and have a better quality of life.

But to achieve better function, we need to understand that abdominals, trained in isolation on a mat, don't improve our functional everyday movements. Most people don't even realize that the abdominal muscles are used throughout the day very naturally, just like all the other muscles. Basic movements like getting up from a chair, standing, bending and walking are supported by the core. If we are not even using our abdominals for our functional needs, of what use is it to yearn for a flat tummy? *Our shape is a by-product of superior function.*

How many of us are familiar with the two layers of abdominal muscles that have completely different functions?

The abdominals comprise inner and outer core muscles.

The inner core muscles include the pelvic floor, transversus abdominis (TrA), internal obliques and diaphragm.

The outer core muscles or the global muscles are also referred to as the 'movers', as they include the superficial abdominal muscles, the back muscles and the hip muscle groups.

The inner core muscles can be imagined as a cylinder that wraps around the entire circumference of the back and stomach. *Activating the inner core as well as the outer abdominal muscles is superior to general abdominal exercises, as when the inner and outer abdominal muscles integrate their functions, spinal stability is maintained.* The muscles of the lower back are also integrated and engaged, thus the whole spine is protected from external loads that may damage the lumbar vertebrae and intervertebral discs.

Most individuals are not aware of the dysfunction that exists as a result of only training the outer abdominal muscles in their workouts. These superficial outer muscles keep compensating for a weak inner core, and the result is a weak and vulnerable lower back. The outer abdominal muscles' (the movers) main function is aiding movement and not stability. Stability is increased by working on inner core muscles only.

To put it simply, if you feel the upper and middle section of your abdominals work and can't feel anything on the lower section of the abdominals, then your abdominal exercises are not contributing to spinal stabilization. Spinal stabilization is of utmost importance in our life, as it helps us avoid overuse of the spine with unnecessary flexion and extension with an active inner core.[15] Our ab exercises will not support our spine in a neutral position while standing, sitting and bending, since the core has not been conditioned to be active or employed during these movements.

You may hear your trainer yell, 'Pull your belly in!' as s/he tries to tell you to stabilize your spine, but there is a gap between understanding and executing these instructions. Detailed below are the two types of core engagements that stabilize, protect and strengthen the back:

- Hollowing/drawing the navel into the spine;
- Bracing the core.

We use both of these techniques in our everyday life for different activities at different times.

Hollowing/Drawing the Navel into the Spine

'Draw in the belly' is a term used a lot nowadays. Sucking the belly button towards the spine helps in activating the transverse abdominis (TrA). *The TrA is a core muscle that is deep and close to the spine, so pre-activation of the TrA before any activity or exercise supports the spine.* As you follow the instructions to appropriately draw in the belly, you will create an intra-abdominal pressure that will make you feel strong, stabilized, confident, self-assured and positive. This is the general feedback from even 80-year-olds who learn this activation! It must be practised while sitting as well as standing, walking and undertaking other activities. When used often, it improves posture and stabilizes the spine in all our activities and movements.

Steps to engage the pelvic floor and TrA:

Step 1: Engaging the TrA first

- Lie down on your back with knees bent.
- Do a few cat-cows by arching the back and then imprinting it. Allow the spine to then relax midway between both extremes. This enables the spine to find its most neutral position. The purpose of this is to allow the natural arch of the lower back to be restored and reset after the effects of bad posture.

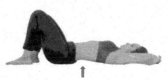
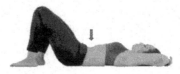

Cat: arching the lower back as high

Cow: imprinting the lower back and pushing it into the floor completely as possible

- Take a deep breath through the nose and expand the abdomen like a balloon without moving the ribcage or the lower back.

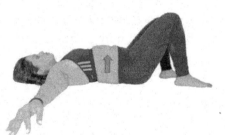

- On the exhalation, imagine the balloon deflating from all sides. Make a slow hissing sound from the mouth as you shrink the abdomen from all sides *without disturbing the natural position of the ribcage and the lower back.*

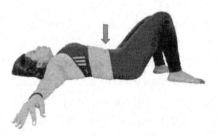

- Core breathing requires the exhalations to be slow and from the mouth, while the inhalations are always through the nose. This breathing is the best way to engage the TrA.
- Imprinting the lower back on the floor or excessively protruding the ribcage will change the natural position of the spine, and the TrA will not get engaged.
- Those who have an excessively flared ribcage, with a large gap between the spine and floor, should push the ribcage down to achieve ideal posture. Core engagement improves posture for those who have excessively flared ribs and excessive lower-back lordosis.

- It is very important to note that drawing in the stomach does not involve rounding the spine either in our abdominal exercises or daily activities.

Step 2: Engaging the pelvic floor

- Visualize squeezing/closing of the urethra and the anus, drawing the pelvic floor upwards. The optimal activation of the core will be when the TrA draws in and the pelvic floor muscles are drawn up simultaneously. But initially, this can be practised in two separate stages. The spine and tailbone must not move while engaging the pelvic floor.
- Hold this engagement and try to breathe.
- Many falter here, as breathing is tricky. Individuals who only know belly breathing find core engagement tough. To get better at this, all you need is practice. *Continuous steady breathing from the ribcage, without inflating and deflating the abdomen, is the only way the core can stabilize your spine.*

By practising just these initial steps, one gets the benefit of stabilizing the spine, immediately priming the body in an ideal posture for any activity or movement, static or dynamic. Yet many make haste and bypass the foundation or think it is just too challenging and don't want to give it a try, thus missing out on a chance to improve their health and the quality of their lives. Don't be intimidated, as the drawing in and bracing technique can be learnt in a practical virtual session with Move Better Wellness in just twenty minutes!

Step 3: Progression to the basic set-up

- The next step would be to bring one arm overhead without changing the position of the rest of the body. The lower back and ribs must not flare. Then, bring the other hand up while maintaining the breath.

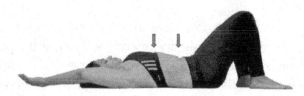

For those who are interested, there are many progressions of the basic set-up that develop strength and accelerate sports performance. You can enrol in a Move Better Programme that helps you achieve your goals.

Core Engagement While Standing, Sitting and Bending

A lot of the workouts today involve repetitive non-functional abdominal exercises. These exercises have little relevance for overall fitness, as they don't contribute to the everyday activities of bending, lifting, carrying weight, stabilization in overhead or rotational movements or enhancing our cardiovascular activities, such as running or cycling. *Performing core exercises and using our core muscles functionally are two different things.* Some individuals may incorporate core exercises in their fitness routines and may be able to perform them very well, but when it comes to functional tasks, the core is completely disengaged. Thus, all the above-mentioned core engagement steps need to be practised while sitting, standing and bending.

Besides standing, walking, sitting and bending, the core must be utilized in squats, lunges and cardiovascular movements.

The core functions 20 per cent while sitting and 40 per cent while standing.

The first step is to always find the neutral position of the spine by performing an anterior and posterior pelvic tilt. After a few repetitions, allow the spine to relax into a position that feels natural. This will be half-way between anterior and posterior tilt. This is a neutral spine, without the distortions created by our unmindful postures. This is similar to lying-down cat-cows. The other steps followed are the same.

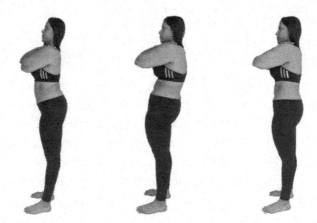

Anterior tilt, posterior tilt and neutral standing
posture with core braced 40 per cent

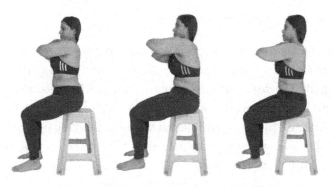

Anterior tilt, posterior tilt and neutral spinal position
while sitting with core braced 20 per cent

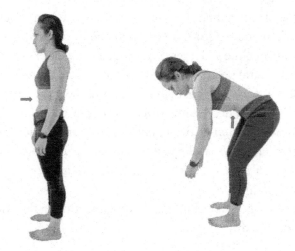

Ideal bending posture with core engagement

First find the neutral spinal position while standing. Engage the core and then hinge. Before you attempt this, refer to page 79 for hinging movements.

Our Buttocks Are Part of the Core

The buttock/glute muscles are part of the core and are a pelvic-lumbar stabilizing muscle, contrary to what many may think. Sitting all day deactivates the glutes. That is why, before we get into advanced forms of exercises, such as loaded squats, dead-lifts and lunges, it is vital that all our stabilizing muscles are highly engaged and active. We must keep squeezing those buttocks as a regular part of our day, either when getting up from the chair or when performing daily tasks such as brushing teeth, bathing, cooking or waiting in queues. 500 squeezes a day will fire that backside, and it will share the load with the other leg muscles when we walk, stand and exercise. Even when you lie down on the stomach or on the back, you can perform glute squeezes. Standing for long hours makes us lose the neutral position of the lower back, and fatigue sets in. A quick buttock squeeze held for a minute works magic, as it resets the spine, decreasing lower disc compression.

The dual action of an employed core from the anterior and an active buttock from the posterior encases and safeguards the spine, which is in the centre. Think of it as a tasty sandwich loaded with life-long perks!

Let's see how the glutes help in stabilization in the bracing technique below.

Bracing Technique

The hollowing technique of core engagement is the base on which the bracing technique can be developed in bending and explosive movements. Some may find this less technical and easier to master.

The steps of the bracing technique are as follows:

- Standing: The bracing technique of core activation is learnt best in a more dynamic posture.
- Spinal position while bracing: It should be noted that changing the shape of the spine into an anterior pelvic tilt or posterior pelvic tilt doesn't stabilize the spine. Maintaining a neutral spinal position helps engage the core and decreases chances of lower-back pain in activities, exercises or movements. Squeezing the glutes at 100 per cent capacity sets the lower back in its natural position effortlessly and primes the body for the challenge. The bracing technique is a boon for people with an anterior tilt, as it engages the glutes while activating the core, which helps the spine stabilize better.
- Activating the core: This form of engagement can be likened to a tightening of the core muscles as an automatic reaction when someone is about to hit you in the stomach. What we instinctively do as a stress response is to stiffen the abdominals to endure the impact. The whole abdomen—upper, lower, as well as the sides—get tighter and firmer. It is not a sucking in of the belly, nor is it fully pushing it outwards. The size of the abdomen stays the same. The pelvic floor muscles are also drawn up in the bracing technique, just as in the hollowing technique.
- Learning to breathe: The automatic reflex on stiffening will be to stop breathing. This is fine as we require more stabilization during the challenging portion of a movement. We can inhale on the easier portions of movement that require less stability of the core. For example, while bending forward, follow the steps to brace

while standing, then hold the breath while you bend and pick up the object from the floor. Once you have picked up the object you can inhale.

Whichever technique one uses, eventually it all boils down to integrating it with our regular movements.

Difference between Hollowing and Bracing

The difference between the hollowing and the bracing techniques lies in the number of muscles used. Bracing involves an engagement of the inner core, outer core, the pelvic floor, diaphragm, as well as the glutes. This is the reason why many may find this technique more effective during exercise, because stabilization utilizes many other global muscles. Obviously, using more muscles is advantageous. This is why many feel that just hollowing might not be enough, especially when it comes to heavy weightlifting, pushing something heavy or doing any other tasks that require spinal protection. If you start a workout with the bracing technique, it is a great way to get you all geared up for action. This stance is the position most athletes use before doing an explosive movement.

Using Both Techniques

Abdominal hollowing brings awareness to the smaller muscle groups and is used for lighter activities such as sitting, standing, walking and picking up light objects. Bracing increases confidence to carry heavier weights and generate power while lifting overhead weights or while picking up something heavy.

On frequent use of the core, one finds that it aids the whole movement chain by increasing stability and strength, while protecting vulnerable body parts from injury. With a weak core, posture and gait are often compromised.

Breath and the Core

Many people have the misconception that yogic breathing is enough. When it comes to stabilizing the spine or pushing yourself in cardiovascular activities, belly breathing is not the most effective option. You cannot belly-breathe while brisk walking. Therefore, we engage the core in a different way for different activities and breathe in a different way for different purposes. *Each breathing technique has its own benefit as well as its limitations. One type of breathing cannot provide all the possible and necessary benefits. Breathing is undoubtedly an important part of movement and brings refinement and ease to movement, provided the technique used is right.* Only then will all movements be coordinated harmoniously. A capable body must know how to continue to breathe efficiently while keeping the core fully activated. A good place to start is with the breathing section below, which develops a good base in 360-degree breathing, after which you will be proficient with core engagement in this section.

A word of caution: If you are a shallow breather or have tightness in the chest and spinal muscles, you might not be very successful in core engagement and might harm yourself in the process.

Skipping the basics and not learning to breathe correctly during the process of core engagement and jumping straight into abdominal and Pilates exercises is undeniably fruitless!

Faulty Core Activation

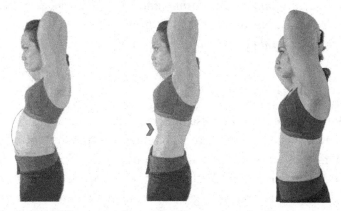

Image 1: A disengaged core leads to a sway back posture and lower back pain
Image 2: An overactive and over engaged upper abdomen leads to respiratory and pelvic floor issues
Image 3: A perfectly engaged core that maintains the integrity of the spine and aids in spinal stabilization

As seen above, it is easy to get into faulty activation techniques, thinking that the abdominals are drawn in. A result of imbalanced workouts is that many draw in the upper abdominals and miss out on spinal stabilization, as the other parts of the abdominals are ignored. *The progress of right core engagement cannot be rushed and should be practised in small doses daily.*

Ill-Effects of Overdoing Abdominal Exercises

Many are obsessed with their core to gain flatter bellies. The TrA should function when it is supposed to; if it is over-contracted, it will disturb its natural function. Overdoing abdominal exercises can lead to an abdomen that is permanently clenched. This will disable the downward movement of the diaphragm, leading to breathing disorders. Another side effect is an uncontrollable leaking bladder, which can result from either a tight pelvic floor or a weak pelvic one. *The cause of the leaky bladder must first be determined, and only then should kegel exercises and pelvic floor exercises be performed.* Some think kegels are important to strengthen their pelvic floor muscles and practise them repeatedly. *But if you don't have any symptoms that suggest you have a weak pelvic floor, you need not take up kegels simply because it's healthy. If we follow the above steps to train our core and use it, it is enough for life-long pelvic health. Moreover, if we take the pains to learn core engagement, it has far superior results than simply performing kegels.* The best way to have a functional TrA is to keep moving throughout the day with an employed core. It will not only give your spine more stability and longevity, but will keep that belly flat!

Bending Better—Hinging

Minal, 60 years of age, resides in Vishakapatnam. She came to me with lower-back and knee pain. She had ten abdominal surgeries at different points in her life that left her intestines and gut in a mess. Besides that, she always felt a lack of confidence in decisions and felt very fearful of many things, including pushing herself in exercises. She learnt and started to practise the above-mentioned core hollowing technique and how to bend/hinge efficiently with the virtual course Move Better Wellness offers. After using these two techniques in all her small daily activities like bending and picking up the phone from the bed, or bending forward daily to brush teeth, she has completely transformed her fitness and health levels as she can now climb stairs and go on hikes which is something she has avoided doing for thirty years!

A young 31-year-old from Ahmedabad came to me with lower-back, shoulder, neck, knee, ankle, calf and foot pain after her second child. Unfortunately, this is very common among young mothers who find themselves out of shape and suffer from multiple aches and pains a few years after childbirth. Rehabilitating the core after C-sections and retraining the body to bend and efficiently pick up your baby with ease is a one-month educational programme Move Better Wellness offers to help women regain their strength and fitness levels.

Nirali had a hysterectomy at 50 and developed hernia due to tucking bedsheets every day. One can suffer needlessly due to poor spinal strength and improper bending habits. Learning how to bend safely is an invaluable boon to prevent yourself from further complications post surgeries and prevent further degeneration for those who have herniated or degenerative discs. Simply follow the steps of how to hinge mentioned below and incorporate them in your daily activities to safeguard your back.

Bending well naturally engages our core and ensures we use it throughout the day. Another term for bending is hinging. A hinge is when there is maximum motion at the hip and minimum motion at the knees. This perfects the ability to separate hip movements from spinal movements by moving only from the hip and not from the back. *The minimum usage of the back and knees while bearing a load is how the hinge protects the lower spinal discs from unnecessary wear and tear and increases longevity. The hinge is the best movement to understand how the pelvis and neck are very much part of the core.*

For optimal mechanics, it is important to first learn to stabilize the spine with the hollowing or bracing technique, learn to breathe right in it and then learn to hip hinge. The spine handles load best when it is set in the most neutral position. If even one part isn't aligned, the way the body distributes load is uneven. Setting the spine in the most efficient position in all movements should be our primary focus. The best way to understand this is a hip hinge. It is the most commonly used posture in everyday tasks, such as lifting things off the floor or other activities that require us to bend forward—for example, tucking in the bedsheet or rearranging things on the lower shelf of a cabinet, opening drawers, lifting our suitcase off the baggage carousel or picking up babies. Detailed below is the ideal way to bend.

- Use a stick that is approximately 3.5–4 feet long and hold it with both hands behind the back.
- With one hand, hold the stick behind the neck and, with the other, support the stick on the tailbone.

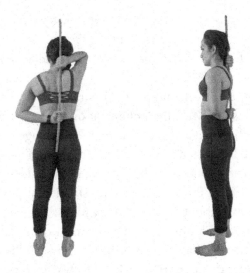

- The rod should maintain contact with your head, mid-back and sacrum and should end at the tailbone. Ensure the stick doesn't protrude beyond the buttocks, as it will clash with the wall. We use the stick to get feedback from the spine to check if it is in a stationary position while performing the hinge.
- Stand 10 inches away from the wall, with the toes pointing forward and feet hip-width apart or slightly wider for a stable base.
- Brace/hollow the core and move forward in a hinge, ensuring all contact points still remain intact. The lower back shouldn't touch the stick, nor should the mid-back be excessively rounded.

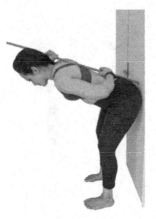

A parallel hinge with maximum range

- The knees shouldn't bend excessively forward but should be parallel to the shin. You should feel a stretch in the buttocks and hamstring.
- Imagine someone pulling your hips back as you lower the trunk and someone pushing the hip forward as you rise. It is important to lead the movement with the hip and not the back as you bend and return to the upright position.
- Always squeeze the glutes after rising.
- If you find you need to move away from the wall or get closer to it, adjust your feet accordingly. The aim is for the buttock to lightly touch the wall with every repetition.
- Once you gain confidence, try doing the same without the help of the stick. Instead of holding the stick, you can let your arms simply hang forward, relaxed.
- Pull the shoulder blades back to keep the upper back active, otherwise it will round out.
- Keep the chin tucked in and don't look up or down; instead, look straight in front of you. The gaze is crucial, as it determines the alignment of the entire spine.

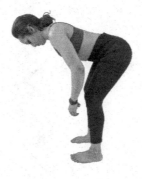

Hinging without the stick

- Depending on your hamstring flexibility, your hinge will decide how far forward your back can go. Greater flexibility in the hip will allow the back to be parallel to the hip. But that isn't important. *It is more important to understand the limit of our personal hinge, as the back will stop moving forward once the hip stops moving backward.*

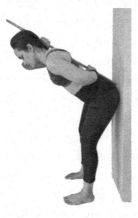

Hinging range on an individual with tight hips and hanstrings

- It is important to coordinate the timing of the whole spine and hip movement. Take the example of a see-saw where both ends are perfectly timed—while one end goes down, the other proportionally rises. This will only happen if we don't dissociate the back from the hip and they synchronize.

Lifting Optimally

While lifting objects in daily activities, you can protect the back by following these steps.

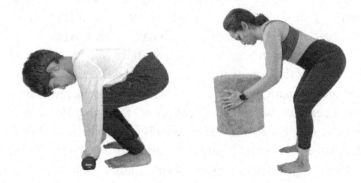

- Depending on how close you are to the object, you can hinge to the maximum and then bend the knees, without altering the spine, to reach the object to be lifted. The knees stay parallel to the shin and don't overshoot the ankle too much. Depending on hamstring flexibility and other factors, individuals have different hinge/hip mobility. Thus, bending the knees helps to reach the object below.

- Before we lift the object, retract (push down) the shoulder blades and grasp the object with both hands in order to avoid a twist in the back.
- Depending on the weight of the object, brace or hollow the core accordingly.
- Lift the object and quickly protect the back by squeezing the glutes.

At Indian weddings, the backs of the new bride and groom are tortured with the customary obligation of touching the feet of all the elders in exchange for blessings. A word of advice: *Perform the hinge instead of bending down and be 'actively impolite' and not inactively polite.* So even if your hinge does not reach the feet, be satisfied with half the blessings!

The prevalence of back pain in India is estimated at 60 per cent of the population, with a higher risk exposure in the female population.[16] If we don't hinge, which is the foundation for a dead-lift, we will never get better at carrying loads. Poor mechanics leads to degenerated discs early in life due to inefficient patterns of lifting and bending all day. Young people fear to perform dead-lifts in their fitness routines, because they feel they will injure the back. Some, in their enthusiasm, get injured and drop out of fitness programmes, as they have no foundational training of the correct mechanics. But few start training the basics first.

Start by correctly hinging to lift a pencil off the floor, then a 1 litre bottle, then a 5 kg knapsack, then finally prime yourself for carrying heavier loads. With every stage, your skill increases your movement confidence. Confidence and good movement go hand in hand. *If you don't apply the foundational movement of a hip hinge, you will never get better at 'other movements', as this is the first step where you learn to 'not use the spine' and preserve its fluidity without compromising it.* We often misinterpret the words, 'You need to have a strong back.' *The spine isn't meant to be strong; it is meant to be supple, and the muscles surrounding the spine are meant to be strong and stable.* The spine cannot preserve its suppleness if it gets damaged through misuse and overuse. It is believed that Joseph Pilates said, 'You are only as old as your spine is flexible.'

Common mistakes of the hinge:

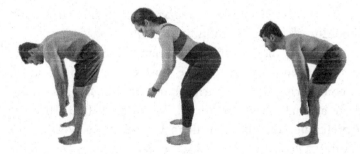

Upper back rounding, lower back excessively curving and head looking up

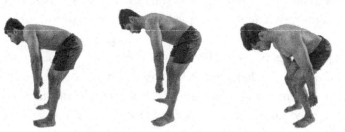

Upper trapezius tensed and shoulder blades disengaged,
feet pointed out and valgus knees

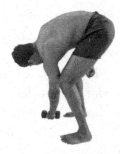

Twisting to pick up object

Sitting Better—Squatting

As many as 1,20,000 knee replacements[17] and 70,000 hip procedures[18] take place in India annually.

Squatting has earned a bad reputation over the years and has been proclaimed to be 'unsafe'. Hence many avoid it, considering it to be harmful and bad for the knees. But these are half-baked theories.[19] [20] [21] In rural India, there is a preference for giving birth in the squatting position for natural deliveries. If we observe babies, the squat is the equivalent of sitting comfortably for them, as they go about their various activities. They start squatting as a natural self-taught movement pattern, which enables them to transition from sitting on the floor to standing. So, if we were all squatting since childhood and were very comfortable in it, what has changed? Why has the avoidance of natural movement patterns become the new norm? *Various reasons are cited for damaged and degenerated knees and backs, but the fountainhead is sedentary culture with inactive glutes, a disengaged core and a lack of mobility and strength.* The introduction of chairs in our modern world has led to the disuse of the deep squat. When we sit on a chair, we condition ourselves with limited mobility. If we use the deep squat, it keeps us supple, as it involves more flexibility and joint mobility as compared to sitting on a chair. *The underuse of the basic squat not only compromises on the skill and mobility required for it, but this lack of skill also reflects in how most choose to sit and get up from a chair.*

The squat will definitely lead to discomfort and pain if we suddenly decide to try it without having the basic requirements—flexibility and mobility. The deep squat isn't bad for us, but getting into squats without good flexibility and mobility is definitely dangerous. *The key is to 'use' the squat in our daily life and not just our fitness.* Most knee problems actually arise because we don't use innate movement patterns that the body is meant for. As Gray Cook writes, 'Nature hasn't made the squat as a loading pattern, but it is more a functional movement pattern used in everyday life that requires mobility.'[22] *Natural movements are used sparingly in fitness, without understanding that the basic human movements like hinging and squatting lead to health and longevity.* We don't generally squat to pick up something heavy from the floor, we hinge. So, it becomes unnecessary to load our squats while exercising, especially if we feel uncomfortable doing a basic bodyweight air squat. But in gyms, we squat with weights and avoid hinges, or our squats look like hinges due to lack of mobility and unskilled training. Thus, in daily functional tasks, the body is confused as it doesn't know how and when to bend and how to sit and get up. *The intelligent body knows when to use a squat and when to hinge, as they have different mechanics and a different purpose.*

How Do We Protect and Strengthen Our Knees to Last a Lifetime?

A lot of controversy revolves around what the ideal knee position should be in daily movements. A common misunderstanding is that 'you should never bring your knees excessively forward' and 'your knees must not overshoot the ankle'. *Without understanding how movement patterns work, we are influenced by these myths and make these specific adjustments and alterations without realizing how that adjustment impacts the whole body!*

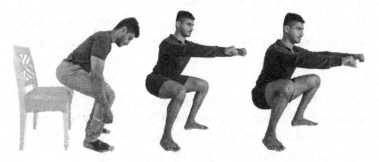

Sitting on a chair, air squat and deep squat

As seen above, sitting on a chair or squatting in the air have the same movement pattern.

A good air squat will visually look like you're sitting on a chair. To get into a deep squat, the knees must naturally overshoot the ankles, since this posture involves the mobility and participation of all the muscles, joints and ligaments of the entire body to balance itself. However, while sitting on a chair, the knees may or may not overshoot the ankles. To sit on a chair with a 90-degree bend in the knees means we have to hinge. As we have learnt earlier, the hinge requires the knees to stack under the ankle. *Thus, for individuals who cannot bring the knees forward, they must perfect the hinge to safeguard the back while sitting on a chair. The hinge will strengthen muscles while maintaining a neutral spinal position.*

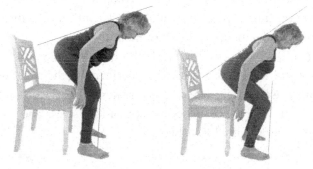

Sitting with a hinge keeping the knees stacked under the ankle and sitting with a squat with the knees slightly overshooting the ankle

Similar to the hinge, safeguarding the spine in squats is vital. You can do this by pushing the knees beyond the ankle. *While the body is suspended in the air during a squat, it is imperative for us to bring the knees forward so we can protect the back. Strengthening our quadriceps (leg) muscles is a non-negotiable as it protects our knees to make them last a lifetime.*

Thus, whether we keep the knees folded at 90 degrees and use the hinge or bring our knees forward in a squat to sit on a chair, it is imperative to be 'skilled' in the hinge and squat in order to protect the back! Most people are not skilled in their hinging mechanics nor at squatting and place their hands on the thighs to support themselves while getting up. There are repercussions to constantly supporting the thighs to sit as well. *If we keep overprotecting our knees, the muscles become weak, making the knee joint a vulnerable spot that will undergo wear and tear even at the slightest impact!* The repetitive support we use while sitting and getting up thus comes with its own baggage. Think of the multiple times a day we sit and get up. Each time, we get an opportunity to strengthen the muscles without exercising, but we still choose comfort! We not only deactivate our muscles during the whole day, but to top this off, we create added stress on the back and knees with our unskilled movements and lack of mobility.

This is what poor squatting techniques look like. All these alterations and adjustments while performing the squat lead to compensations elsewhere. This creates unequal load on the knee joint, wearing it out sooner with added stress and strain that degenerates the lower back.

Compromises in squats can be seen as below:

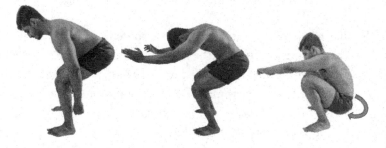

Image 1: Knees behind and back forward: shows a lack of quadricep strength and a tight, overused back. This will eventually degenerate the lower back and weaken the knees.
Image 2: Rounded upper back indicates a lack of hip, ankle and posterior chain mobility.
Image 3: Not being able to go into a deep squat without a posterior pelvic tilt due to lower ankle mobility and or anatomical restrictions. As a mobility position this is not harmful but in a loaded squat this can compromise the lower back.

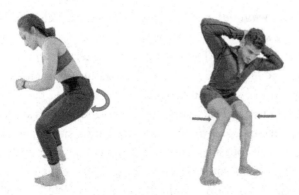

Image 1: Getting into a posterior pelvic tilt too early due to tight hamstrings can lead to degeneration in the lower back with repetitive movement.

Image 2: Valgus knees (knees caving inward) while performing a squat is a sign of weak glutes which can damage knees over a period of time.

When we sit/squat or hinge/bend, the muscles in the trunk stabilize the spine; the glutes, quadriceps and hamstrings bear the load. The whole posterior chain and the ankles and quadriceps of the anterior chain need to be mobile for right alignment. Muscles that are inactive and tight interfere with natural loading patterns, and we add to this by not allowing the knees to move over the ankles and bear weight on the quadriceps. So what happens instead? The burden of the whole body is borne by the poor spine! The back is tight and overused because of all these unnatural manipulations. This is why back problems are followed by knee problems and vice versa.

It is not a one-time movement that is responsible for damage to the knees and the lower back; instead, it is dis-use of the quadriceps over a period of time that's responsible for it. *It is important to know what to move and what not to, what to use and what not to use.* Strength must be developed slowly to sit and stand without support, in perfect alignment. It can be done at any age. The more we use external supports, the weaker and less mobile we become, making us dependent and losing confidence in movement.

After knee and back surgeries, many individuals are scared to perform squats or bend. But there isn't a single person, be it with or without surgeries, that I haven't encouraged to do some degree of a squat or a hinge, as these are the most basic and natural functions of the human body. We cannot live without them! *Even if you are sitting on a chair, it is a half squat! Think of how many times pre- or post-surgery, with or without bad knees, you are repeatedly sitting and getting up from a chair! How many squats a day is that? If you are doing it wrong, you are still harming those knees, with or without surgery!* You can prevent or postpone surgery for half worn-out knees, provided you don't wear them out quickly by loading them incorrectly.

How to align our ankles and knees with the spine so we can safely align our bones to distribute loads evenly is the skill that we have forgotten. Even after surgeries, we can enjoy the freedom of natural movement that has become taboo due to theories of how bending and squatting are bad for health. Yes, they are bad! But only if you are performing them badly! The same thing done right can be liberating.

The squat is the most widely used position to assess athletes as well as non-athletes for strength and mobility, because it exposes weakness and tightness in a person immediately. It is a great way to check your mobility in the feet, ankles, calves, hamstrings, glutes and all the spinal muscles as well as the shoulder. Without a mobility programme, it is tough to get into and maintain good squatting mechanics.

Using the mobility squat

Mobility squats against the wall are a good way to start learning to squat. It is also a test to expose the areas that are constricted. It is a great warm-up, pre-fitness exercise and can be used for developing a good squatting technique, as it teaches us the correct alignment of the back and knees.

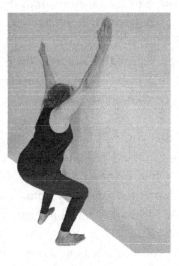

- Turn your face towards a wall.
- Keep the feet apart slightly wider than your hips.
- Keep the feet pointing forward with the toes approximately 4 inches away from the wall. Then turn them slightly outward.

- Hold your hands up in a 'V' shape, with the thumbs facing back.
- Raise the arches of the feet by turning the kneecaps slightly outward to align them with the third toe.
- Lower into a squat while keeping the knees slightly wider than the ankles.
- Bear the body weight on the heel.
- Allow your knees to move forward. Allow the chest and head to come forward as far as possible. The edge of the palm must touch the wall. Don't keep the back very straight; allow it to lean forward into the wall. You will reach a point where you will feel like you are about to fall backward. That is where you will stop.
- Come up and repeat this multiple times. Each day you may be able to go lower than the previous with a natural increase in overall mobility.

On attempting this you will be able to gauge the extent of tightness in your upper back, shoulders, mid and lower back, glutes, hips, hamstrings, quadriceps, ankles and calves. Regular practice of these mobility squats, combined with soft-tissue release in Chapter 6 will improve flexibility of the muscles. You will definitely be going deeper in those squats, pain-free with a protected back and knees. Many individuals have delayed and averted surgery despite having conditions like knock knees and bunions. Superior movement skills reduce the wear and tear and degeneration and help preserve our joints to last us a lifetime.

Optimal way of sitting and getting up from a chair

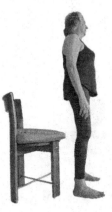

1. Stand with the feet pointed forward hip-width apart or even slightly wider.
2. Align the knees slightly wider than the ankle while grounding the big toe and the entire foot into the floor.

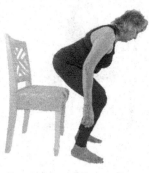

3. Push the buttocks back while grounding the heels into the floor as you lower the body.

4. Allow the knees to come naturally as far forward as they can so the back is unmoved.

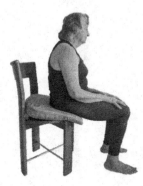

5. Make sure you are not in a posterior pelvic tilt sitting on the tailbone.

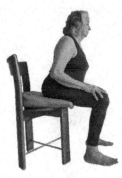

6. We sit on the sit-bone* and not the tailbone.

_____

* The sit–bone/sitz bone or ischial tuberosity are the two bones under the buttocks which absorb our body weight when we sit.

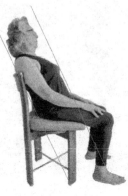

7. The central idea is to maintain a neutral arch of the lower back when we transition from standing to sitting. This must be maintained even if we lean back into the chair. Leaning back with rounded shoulders alters our spinal curvature.

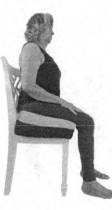

8. To make sitting effortless without any back support, I recommend using a wedge cushion that elevates the spine.

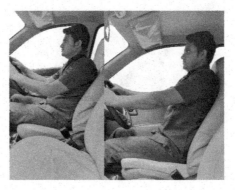

9. Flight and car seats are sunk in, pushing the spine into a posterior pelvic tilt.[23] This might remind you of the times you just couldn't get up after sitting on a low sofa or you began to limp after getting off a long flight or car journey. Make this cushion your best friend and carry it with you wherever you go.

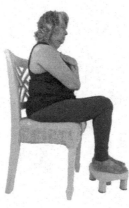

10. The golden rule of sitting should be that your knee should never be higher than the hip.

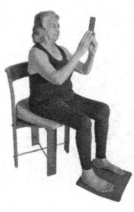

11. Sometimes, because of the height of the chair, we can't place the feet comfortably on the floor. So, we rest our feet on an object that fills up the gap between the foot and the floor. Make sure you maintain a higher hip-to-knee ratio.

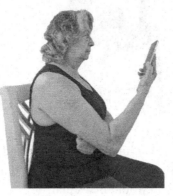

12. Any gadgets used like the computer, phone or while reading a book should be at eye level.
13. The shoulder should always be externally rotated.

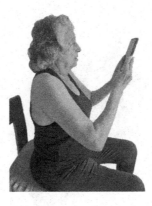

14. The arms and elbows should be kept at the proper height so they don't elevate the upper trapezius.

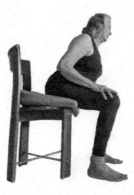

15. While getting up, place the feet hip-width apart, ground the heels, rotate the knees outward and drive up from the glutes, like you would in a squat.

16. Leaning forward while getting up should not alter the position of the back. Leaning forward is fine as long as the

spinal curvature remains unchanged, taking help from the core that stabilizes the spine.

17. After standing, always squeeze the glutes to release any compression in the lower back.

Climbing Better—Lunge

The lunge is a functional movement we use when we lower ourselves to sit on the floor. You may also use the lunge position to tie your shoelaces or accomplish tasks similar to squats, like rearranging things on the lower shelves. If we don't practise lunges, nor sit on the floor daily using a lunge, we lose the ability to do so with time. Forward lunges help us if we ever have to take large strides and step over an obstacle. How many times have we hesitated to cross a pile of faeces or an open gutter? Think of the confidence you will have if you can stride over and make it to the other side untainted! Those who perform lunges periodically find an ease in climbing movements such as hiking, climbing a slope or simply getting in and out of a high car. Because lunges are unilateral compared to squats, it is easier for us to detect problems in one knee as compared to the other. It is also simple for us to determine our individual leg strength and work on reducing the difference between the two. There are two types of lunges: the split lunge and the true lunge.

Split Lunge and True Lunge

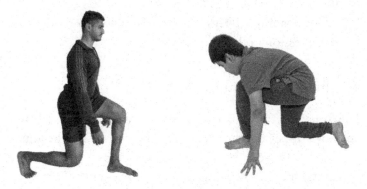

Use of a split lunge (knee stays parallel to the ankle) while sitting and
getting up from the floor

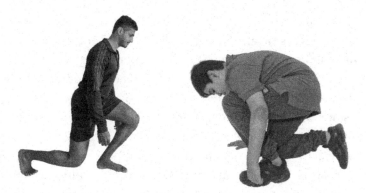

Everyday tasks like tying shoe laces can involve a true lunge
(knees beyond the ankle)

Both methods can be adopted depending on what our knees
can handle, but the true lunge is superior to the split lunge,
as it primes the body for more functional movements like
squatting and climbing stairs. This is because it loads the

quadriceps muscles and keeps the ankles mobile. If you do not have any knee pain, it is good to challenge yourself with the true lunge. Many feel their knee hurts when it is pushed forward beyond the ankle. Some also experience pain after a certain point in their lunge. Their movement range is limited, and they can't lower the back knee completely to the floor. We cannot abstain from this all our lives, since sitting on a chair and stepping on and off different surfaces will require the knee to sometimes overshoot the ankle. Sitting and getting up from the floor effortlessly also requires the full range of the lunge. Rather than curbing our natural functional abilities, we must try to troubleshoot so we can live in freedom rather than living over-cautiously. We can perform soft-tissue releases and stretches as shown in Chapter 6, to remove any soft tissue restrictions that can be a cause of knee pain. We then re-test to see if the movement feels better.

Knee Position in Squatting and Lunging

Training the knee forward in a true lunge can be done with the help of a wall.

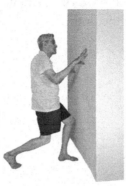

- Touch the toes to a wall and align both your legs under the hip.
- Slide one leg behind. If the gap between the legs is too narrow, you won't be able to lower yourself comfortably, and if the distance is too much, the front knee will not go beyond the ankle.
- The back toes must point forward and must be firmly grounded. Lift the heel off the floor. If the sole of your foot is tight, or your toes are not mobile, this will not feel comfortable, and the back leg will not provide balance and steadiness.
- Place the hands on the wall and bend both knees simultaneously, with the front knee touching the wall.
- The weight of the front leg rest on the heel, and the weight of the back leg on the toes.
- While lowering the body, the back must be straight, distributing the body weight equally on both legs.
- Don't go too low if your knee hurts.
- First develop strength in the glutes and core and improve mobility by using the techniques in the squat section. Only then will it be easy to push the lunge deeper, and be comfortable with the back knee completely on the floor.

Difference in Knee Positions in the Hinge, Squat and Lunge

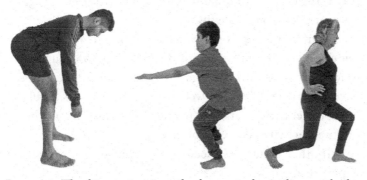

Image 1: The hinge requires the knees to be in line with the ankle, with shins kept vertical. So when we pick up a load, we protect our knees and back, as our bones are aligned and stacked one on top of the other.

Image 2: A squat, however, will be compromised if the knees don't go forward. We cannot prevent the knee moving forward, as we will start compensating with the back.

Image 3: The lunge is a loading pattern that gives us the flexibility to keep the knee in line with the ankle or overshoot it to suit our needs. It is the safest way to rehabilitate the lower extremities, as it is versatile.

Using Daily-life Loading Patterns More than Dysfunctional Ones

'Functional training' has been coined as a fitness fad that delivers fancy cardiovascular exercises. We must understand that functional exercises are the ones that mirror the moving patterns that we use in everyday life. Our everyday functional movements must be prioritized when we spend our valuable time on fitness. If I am given a choice between a split lunge and a true lunge, I would obviously opt for the one that gives me more functional benefits.

Even if we are doing yoga or Pilates daily, we must understand that neither conditions our back to lift up heavy weights or condition our legs to climb stairs efficiently. We have to actually lift heavy weights and climb stairs regularly to get better at them and not presume that our current choice of fitness activity takes care of them.

Another instance is seen when a person opts to sit on a quadriceps machine in the gym and avoid hinges, squats and lunges. The machines used in gyms build isolated muscle strength, not functional strength that uses multiple muscles and conditions the body in stability and motor control. The body only adapts to the loads we train it in and use most of the day. Machines in the gym are a good way for an elderly person or beginner to start, but as strength builds up, one must train the body in all the foundational movements. *We will never get the rewards of our fitness if we avoid the very patterns of movement that are inescapable in everyday life.*

How to Climb Stairs

The mechanics of climbing stairs are similar to a leg stance implemented while lunging forward.

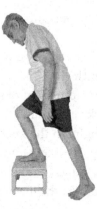

- While climbing up, always land on the heel first or full foot and not the toe.
- After placing the heel, align the knee with the third toe.
- Lean the body weight forward and use the heel of the leading leg to lift the body. This helps, especially if the riser of the staircase is high. Using the heel protects the knee from impact. As long as your bodyweight is on the heel, even if the knee overshoots the ankle slightly, it is safe. People with knee pain can climb stairs without apprehension in this manner.
- Always use alternate legs while climbing so you don't tire out and overuse one leg.

Climbing down stairs is tricky for individuals with knee pain. Certain measures need to be taken to comfortably climb down without pain. Consider some professional guidance with a practical course with us to guide you through this journey pain-free.

Follow these steps when climbing down:

- Before you step down, make sure the feet and knees are stacked right under the hip.
- Use the toes of the leading foot to step down.
- If you keep the back very straight, there is more impact of our whole bodyweight on the knees. Therefore, push the buttock behind slightly like a hinge. The back will move slightly forward as you suspend the leading foot in the air.
- As you transit to land on the toe of the front foot, the back leg bears the weight on the heel.
- If you are implementing these instructions right now, you will have already noticed the amount the back knee has to bend beyond the ankle to climb down. If you do not first condition the knees to move forward in lunges, you won't feel ease in climbing down.
- The knee of the back leg must line up with the third toe to ensure perfect alignment of the bones.
- As you land completely with the front foot, the back foot lifts off on the toes. Flexibility in the sole of the foot is a prerequisite here, just as in the lunge.

Balancing

'I have sprained my ankle multiple times on occasion. I wear high heels often at night,' said Pariniti, a 28-year-old from Delhi. It is only after her knee started buckling that that she got scared and decided to strengthen her ankle using the methods shared in this section.

Good balancing is an indispensable ingredient prevalent in all movements. The habitual use of balance in everyday movements reduces knee, ankle and hip injuries and prevents falls.[24] It simplifies the mechanics of our squats, hinges, lunges and stair-climbing. It enhances your ability to pre-empt your distance in space while striding or leaping forward. *Assuming children are good at balancing is an incorrect assumption. It is a skill that we exercise when we are young and refine as we grow older.* If we have not trained our ability to balance flawlessly from childhood, we need to incorporate this aspect in our everyday training. Many 80-year-olds visit me only to increase their confidence in balancing. As people age, the lack of confidence in movement is more due to a lack of skill in balancing, which was never developed while they were young.

I have asked some children to balance. Those who have not developed the ability falter. Balancing is also a skill just like other skills, which needs to be trained, till we feel confident we can balance ourselves effortlessly in any circumstance, at any age, with any incapacity. Research verifies that training balance improves overall athletic preparation, as it is crucial for runners. In sports training, long-term balance exercises reduce the risk of injury. Balancing helps postural control in youth and older adults and improves functional activities in daily living.[25]

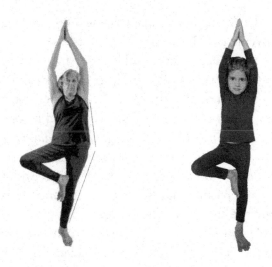

Balancing with a weak *glute medius* makes the hip jut out which creates
unequal load on the feet and knees wearing them out faster

Let's break down this simple balance, the 'tree pose'. Many
may think they are balancing well and can hold the pose for
an entire minute without falling, but they are unaware of the
flaws in the position and compensations taking place while
doing so. As we see in the picture above, the hip juts out to
one side. This exposes weakness in the glute, which doesn't
support the body's weight on one leg efficiently and transfers
the load to the knees and ankle. Balancing with this flaw will
damage the knees instead of strengthening them. Our core
and glutes must work together to brace us while balancing.

Similar misalignment is seen in the squat, lunge and
hinge when a *weak gluteus medius*[26] (one of the glute muscles)
doesn't allow the knees to align themselves over the third toe
in a squat and lunge. This can be observed either in just one
leg or both legs.

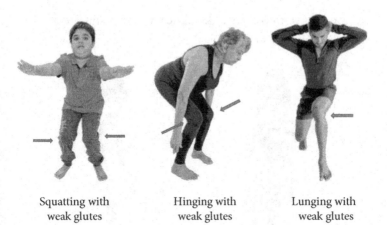

| Squatting with weak glutes | Hinging with weak glutes | Lunging with weak glutes |

Many individuals don't feel their glutes in squats, lunges or while bending. They only burn out the thighs. This is why their performance in walking, running, climbing stairs, hiking cannot be pushed beyond a point. It is too much of a load just for one muscle to bear. Incorporating glute strengthening into your routine even for healthy individuals increases performance, as the burden is equally distributed among all muscles.

The main criteria in any movement pattern are balance, stability and power, which are driven by the centre—the pelvis. Thus pelvic stability and strength are crucial for protecting us from sacroiliac joint dysfunction. Incorporating glute exercises into our regimen refines all our movements.

The Elements of Balance

Balancing is simple, but balancing well can be challenging if we want to meet all the standards of perfection. The glute and core must maintain pelvic–lumbar stability. Aligning the hips while balancing is a sign of a strong and stable pelvis. Raising the arches and not allowing the ankle to drop is mandatory if we want to stabilize the ankle, knee and hip and stack them well under each other.

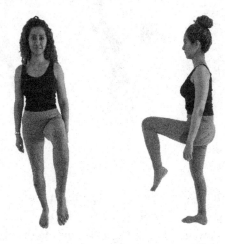

- Bring one leg up till the knee is in line with the hip and hold it for a minute.
- To make balancing easy, we must spread apart the toes, raise the arch and ankle by grounding the big toe and creating a force towards the outer edge of the feet. If your arches or ankles don't collapse, simply spreading the toes is enough.
- Rotate the knee outward so it stays stacked well under the ankle and hip. Don't hyper-extend the knee.
- The core should be engaged naturally and not tucked in a posterior pelvic tilt or an anterior tilt.
- The shoulders should be rolled back with the gaze straight ahead. You will find it impossible to get better at balancing if the eyes are looking up, down or sideways.
- Use the support of a wall with one finger initially to help maintain balance for a minute. You can cautiously remove the finger and try to balance without support. Use it again if you feel unsteady.

This balance strengthens injured ankles and helps create stability in the ankle joint for those who keep twisting it and are susceptible to sprains. Once the above balance is perfected, one should try to increase the challenge by adding some instability to the surface by placing a cushion on the floor. Try balancing on different textured surfaces like grass, sand, mud and pebbles to see what challenge it presents to your feet and ankles. Balancing on varied surfaces is the surest way of becoming adept at facing any movement challenge. Not raising the arch and dropping the ankle or dropping one hip results in a misaligned pelvis.

The common errors that are not taken into consideration while balancing are:

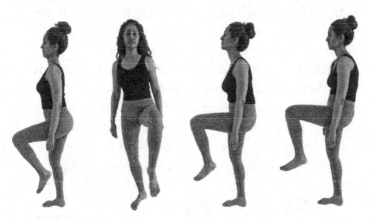

Image 1: Balancing with an excessive anterior tilt and not maintaining proper spinal positions

Image 2: Balancing with feet turned outward and not pointed forward

Image 3: Thrusting the neck forward

Image 4: Rounding the upper back and drooping the shoulders or getting into a posterior pelvic tilt

Pulling and Pushing

I once visited a radiologist, whose arm was tired by the evening. I recall him asking if he could rest his hand on me while taking the sonography. Any other woman would have thought he was a pervert, but understanding where he was coming from, I asked him, 'What are you doing about your arm pain?' The anticipated answer was, 'Nothing'. An anaesthetist who came to me also faced similar issues. *Many people might infer that these are occupational hazards, but in truth our body isn't primed to enjoy the life we want to lead.* Women want toned arms but can't open a heavy door. How can one push themselves towards their fitness goals if the upper limbs can't handle physical challenges of daily life? With today's sedentary culture, shoulder pain, cervical spondylosis, migraines, vertigo, upper-back pain are very common, as they are all products of stiff, unstable and weak upper-back mechanics.

Lack of postural awareness, along with weak back muscles, keeps the shoulder in internal rotation through the day. The shoulder joint doesn't naturally sit in its capsule, and we use and abuse it in compromised positions during all our activities all day long. *Internal rotation of the shoulder becomes the source of a majority of the upper-limb problems we face today.*

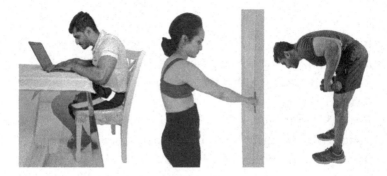

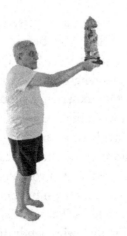

Our desk-bound rounded shoulders lead to an internal rotation of the shoulder which is carried forward in other daily activities such as opening doors, exercising or while grabbing something from the cupboard

Our desk-bound internally rotated shoulders are the same posture we use for basic activities, such as carrying bags and heavy laptops, pulling and pushing doors, grabbing something overhead from a cupboard or storing a suitcase in the overhead cabin of a plane. During our exercises, we use the same incorrect form in push-ups, rows and overhead movements.

When we hinge to lift heavy objects from the floor, the upper-back muscles need to stabilize, otherwise the lower back often bears the brunt of the effort and pays a price. The spine runs all the way from the tailbone to the neck, which makes *the glutes the core of the lower body and the t-spine (thoracic spine) the core of the upper body.*

The common shape we hold most of the day, i.e. with rounded shoulders, is a sign of an inactive and unstable t-spine. The feeling of the muscles of the upper back functioning in basic activities comes as a surprise to many, as they have never felt those muscles work before. When a desk-bound individual starts fitness activities by excessively using pushing movements and chest strengthening exercises such as push-ups, bench presses, etc., they experience shoulder, elbow, neck and upper-back pains, tears and sprains.

The muscles involved in pushing movements are the chest, shoulders and triceps. These chest muscles are already tight from sitting all day with a rounded back and internally rotated shoulders. Loading them further with a tight thoracic spine only invites problems. The same stress pattern is seen in a house-bound individual, who bends down in the kitchen all day, slouches to text and sits on furniture that creates a curve in the spine that makes shoulder problems inevitable. Those who have suffered rotator cuff and labral tears, shoulder impingements and tendinitis know that it takes these injuries months to heal, and trying to avoid using the arm to aid the healing process becomes a nightmare.

To protect our joints from wearing out, we need to reposition our shoulder joint by starting with more pulling movements that strengthen the back, in comparison to pushing ones, which tighten the chest. Even if we have a good weekly workout schedule, the ill-effects of posture during our waking hours makes certain areas in the upper back stiff.[27] Shefali from Indore came to me with kyphosis. The hump on her back was getting worse, and she couldn't find anyone who could correct this for her permanently. This started increasing neck and shoulder pain. Just by following the exercises mentioned below, she was able to rid herself of neck and shoulder pain.

People with tight shoulders, who are missing end range shoulder mobility, start stretching the shoulders in vain.

Tight shoulders are not linked to the shoulder joint. We need to know what is actually causing the problem—it is the tight upper back. Stretching the shoulder will only increase hyper mobility and create an unstable shoulder joint.

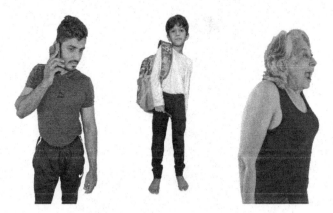

Talking on the phone, carrying a bag and shouting at someone with tense upper trapezius

The upper trapezius is a place where many individuals store their stress and emotion. It is overactive and involved in all the actions of the upper limbs, which makes it feel tight for most people. Tension headaches and shoulder pain are just a few symptoms of tight upper trapezius. *Releasing the tension in the upper trapezius by regular massage gives a lot of relief. But by not strengthening the surrounding muscles, it falls back into its old habit of being overused, thus becoming tight again. Many people are trapped in this cycle of pain that reoccurs every now and then without a permanent solution.*

The muscles that aid in scapula stability or rather controlled mobility are the upper/middle/lower trapezius and the rhomboids and serratus anterior, so strengthening them is non-negotiable.

Exercise 1: Standing rows

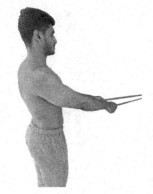

- Use a resistance band and stand with both arms held out in front, shoulder level, with a little tension in the band.

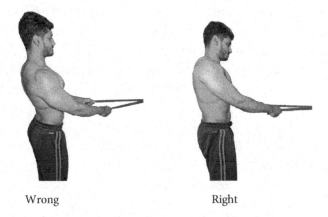

Wrong   Right

- Engage the core so you don't overextend the lower back.

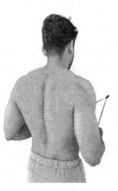

- Depress (push downward) the shoulder blades. This should feel like a stretch for the chest without over-extending the thoracic (puffing the chest out).

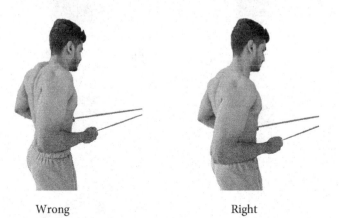

Wrong   Right

- Do not elevate the upper trapezius
- Draw the arms in no more than waist level and feel the upper- and mid-back muscles squeeze.
- Ensure the shoulder is externally rotated while you repeat the exercise twenty-five times.

This basic exercise habituates the shoulder to externally rotate in all our movements.[28] It also helps relieve neck pain. Internal rotation of the shoulder over long periods of time eventually causes shoulder damage.

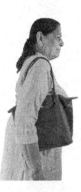

Wrong

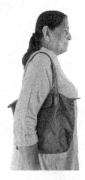

Right (by externally rotating the shoulder)

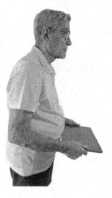

Wrong

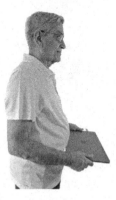

Right (ensuring the shoulders are externally rotated

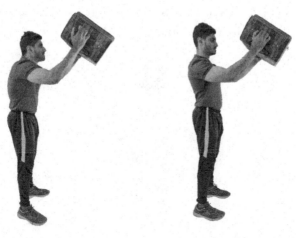

Wrong   Right (Externally rotating the
                                shoulders while grabbing or
                                storing overhead objects)

Externally rotating the shoulder sets the ideal position for the shoulder joint, which is safe when it comes to loading patterns.

Exercise 2: Lower trapezius strengthening

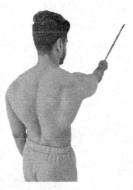

- Loop a resistance band over the door or on a curtain rod, keeping both ends loose.

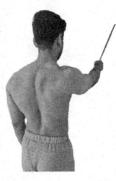

- Hold the loose ends in one hand with a protracted shoulder. Then retract (push down) the shoulder blade. Release the arm and repeat twenty-five times.
- Ensure you don't tighten or use the upper trapezius and focus on the lower trapezius.

This exercise reconditions the upper trapezius to relax and become less dominant in activities, as it strengthens the lower trapezius over time. If you have stress and neck pain, this exercise will make you feel light and relaxed.[29]

Exercise 3: Scapular push-up

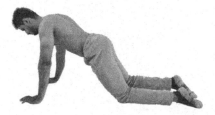

- Kneel down on the floor or bed in a half push-up position or use the quadruped position.

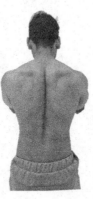

- Lower the shoulder blades and feel them meeting each other.

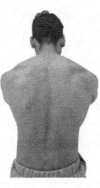

- Then push those shoulder blades apart without rounding the upper back.

- The key is not to move the rest of the body and focus just on the shoulder blades.
- You may want to bend the elbows, but try to keep the arms straight.

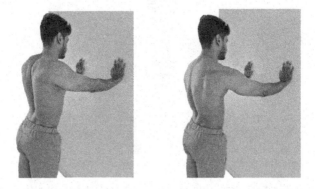

- If this is too tough, you can try it by keeping the arms straight against a wall. Touch the shoulder blades together, then push them apart.
- Do fifteen repetitions of this exercise.

> This exercise helps in T-spine stability and controlled mobility as it activates the scapula. This enables the scapula-stabilizing musculature to perform in upper-torso movements. If you experience upper- and mid-back fatigue and find that hunching your back is unpreventable, then this is the exercise for you.[30]

Exercise 4: Rotator cuff strength

- Tie one end of a light resistance band to a doorknob.

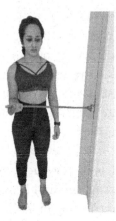

- Stand with one hand facing the door knob and hold the loose end of the band in the opposite hand with the palm facing up.
- Keep the wrist straight and the elbow pushed into the waist.

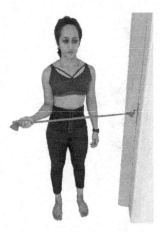

- Move the forearm out.

- Walk away from the door.
- Hold this position for a minute. You will feel an intense burn in the shoulder. If you can't sustain it for a minute, start slowly walking towards the door to reduce the amount of resistance until you can last the entire minute.
- After the minute is up, rotate the arm in a circular motion to ease it out, as it may feel jammed.

Exercises 2 and 3 prep the back muscles, and Exercise 4 strengthens the rotator cuff and helps reduce shoulder pain. When combined with the mobility routine suggested in Chapter 6, these exercises decrease pain, improve posture, increase performance in the torso and add longevity to your shoulder.[31] These exercises work well even as a warm-up routine before you get into fitness activities.

Exercise 5: Shoulder stability

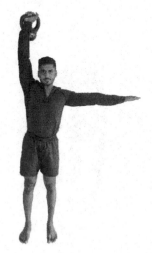

This exercise is a test and is performed to increase shoulder stability. Stabilizing the shoulder joint is imperative, as it helps prevent injuries from overhead movements. If you are placing heavy objects on the top shelf of a cupboard or lifting your cabin baggage from the aircraft, then you need strong and stable shoulders. Strength in the shoulder joint is necessary, and so is stability, which is different. You may have the strength for a certain movement, but does the joint feel stable if the load is heavy? Try this test to see if both your shoulders are strong and stable.

Choose the heaviest weight you can carry overhead with your dominant arm and walk for a minute. Then switch the arms and repeat. If one arm is really stable and can sustain holding the weight but the other arm feels unstable, weak or awkward and gives up much sooner, there is work needed.

As discussed before, many sports cause the overuse one limb as compared to the other. We always have one side slightly stronger than the other, which is the way we are designed. Similarly, certain muscles on the right and left side of the body can be weaker or stronger, depending on use and overuse. *Our job is to maintain a healthy balance between both sides of the body by eliminating vast differences or inequality between them.*

The same applies for the lower limbs. Those who have already tried the lunge on both legs must have discovered the dissimilarity in both sides by now. This means one should incorporate into our fitness routine more exercises that strengthen both sides of the body individually. The rule is to always start with the weaker side. It decides how much the stronger side should do. Often, the weaker side might not be able to function, because there is an underlying mobility issue, not a strength issue.

The human body and its mechanics are complex, so using all the exercises in the mobility programme (Chapter 6) and not eliminating parts of it will take care of most of the underlying issues that an average individual needs to remain mobile. The next step is to develop the ideal posture by strengthening and stabilizing the body by using the foundational movements. This is the right way to approach this programme.

Rotational Stability and Strength

Simple, everyday life movements require some rotational capability, like when you are picking up things from a trolley and placing them in your car, turning around to look over your shoulder to answer phones or rotating to pick up the toothbrush from one side. We need adequate mobility to support rotational movements so that the trunk is able to rotate while twisting to fetch something from the back of the car seat, walking, running, kicking a ball or playing a sport. A capable body is able to take a movement through the full range of motion and generate power while being stable in that position. Visualize a perfect golf shot or a footballer drawing their leg back to shoot at a well-executed goal—a perfect blend of mobility, stability and strength.

Rotational movements require all these three elements and the skill to perform them. If any of these components are lacking, lower disc degeneration is the first effect. You can then predict the long list of injuries and joint degeneration that follow. The abdominal muscles are meant to support and stabilize the lower back while the musculature and joints facilitate twisting and turning in activities that require us to rotate. The foremost cause of disc herniation and slipped disc is the way we bend and then twist to lift things every day. *Rotational movements may look easy, but biomechanically, they involve many muscles. Therefore, it is essential to increase our competence to stabilize the spine as well as constantly work on mobility.*

The Neck

Another element disregarded in rotational movements is our neck. The neck is very much a part of the spine and the core. As we have seen in optimal standing alignment as well as hinging, the neck and core muscles support each other and work in synchronicity to stabilize the body in movement. It is the same with rotational movements. If your neck is out of place, the centre of gravity shifts while rotating, making the movement slipshod.

Our eyes play an important part in neck alignment. The neck follows the direction of the gaze. Some people tend to look to one side while thinking. Unknowingly, doing this for many years makes one side of the neck short and tight while the other is lengthened and overstretched, leading to lopsidedness. While taking passport photographs, many must have experienced the photographer saying, 'Keep your head straight!' Our version of straight often doesn't match his.

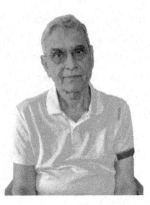

Lopsided neck

You can self-correct this easily using the exercises below.

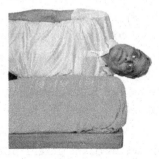

- Lie down on one side of the bed with the shorter side
  on top and the lengthened side below. Stretch in this
  position for a minute. Then reposition your head to
  neutral.

The neck releases (refer to Chapter 6, page 168–171) can also
be done by people who want to get rid of neck discomfort,
pain or a strain. Similarly, if we are gazing at something lower

than eye level, the chin pops out causing the forward head posture. The exercise below strengthens the deep neck flexors.

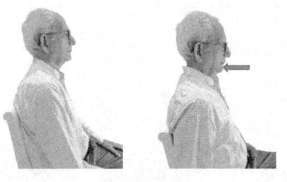

Seated chin tucks

- In a sitting position, push the chin behind. Hold for twenty seconds and then release.
- This can be done lying down on the floor or sitting against a wall.

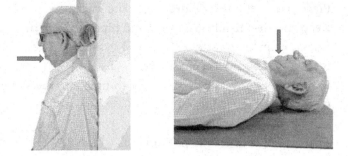

Image 1: Individuals with forward head posture can use the wall for chin tucks. Adjust the gap between the head and the wall with a towel so as to align the spine.

Image 2: Chin tucks performed while lying down on a hard surface

Rotational exercises are also beneficial for individuals with neck, upper- or lower-back pain, as it releases the thoracic and the para-spinal muscles.

Standing Rotations

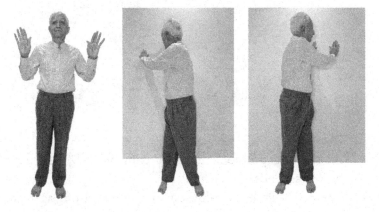

- Stand with your back against a wall.
- Place your feet one foot away from the wall.
- Keep your feet firmly grounded and hip-width apart.
- Rotate your torso to touch the wall behind on one side, with both the palms at chest level.
- Repeat this on the other side. Try to maintain the same placement of the palms on the wall as you rotate on both sides.
- Ensure that your feet do not move as you rotate.
- Do at least ten rotations every day.

You may find one side slightly tighter than the other, but this slowly eases out with daily repetitions.

Seated Chair Rotations

If the wall rotations are fairly easy, then progress to chair rotations for increased mobility.

- Sit at the edge of a chair with the feet firmly grounded on the floor, hip-width apart.
- Place an object between the thighs like a cushion or yoga block and squeeze it so your pelvis is stable.

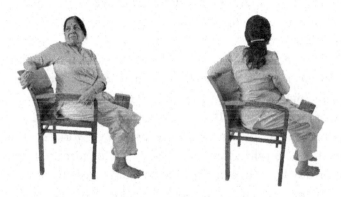

- Turn around to one side without moving the feet. Grip the backrest of the chair with both hands while keeping the spine straight.
- Repeat this on the other side. You should be able to perform this with ease on both sides.
- Neither the feet nor pelvis should shift as you rotate for ten sets.

The standing rotations are facilitated through the pelvis, but the seated rotations remove the pelvis from the equation, thereby increasing mobility.

Breathing Better

Breathing is the most nutritious and subtle function of the body that sustains us. We undermine and take for granted the power of the breath, which has the capacity to either calm us and regulate the body or create chaos.

Let's take a breathing test to find out how efficient our baseline breathing is.

Simply look at the watch and time how many breaths you take in a minute. Anything that is above 10–12 breaths a minute is a sign of anxiety, stress and overload that the body has to deal with.

As we become aware of our breath, it slows down a little, so our usual breathing volumes, when left unchecked, are slightly higher. We must try to achieve a spontaneous breath rate of 10 or less than 10 breaths per minute. Breathing large volumes of air makes the entire body overwork, creating added stress on all its functions in addition to the mental stress we already have. Imagine the havoc that is created within us as our metabolism, circulation, digestion, assimilation and evacuation are all affected. Breathing has a direct impact on our cardiac, digestive, excretory system as well the endocrine and nervous systems.

Inefficient breathing is linked to an array of health problems. *Just like too much food, too much air messes up the whole body's function.* Inhaling too much air reduces our tolerance to carbon dioxide. All of us already have 95–99 per cent oxygen in our red blood cells. The use of oximetres has educated most during the COVID-19 pandemic about maintaining oxygen levels. But it is not the amount of oxygen in the blood cells that is required for our muscles, organs and tissues to be energized. Instead, it has more to do with the amount of carbon dioxide in our blood.

When we retain carbon dioxide in the lungs, it increases the blood pH level, allowing haemoglobin to bind more tightly to oxygen. Being more soluble than oxygen, carbon dioxide readily diffuses into the red blood cells[32] and allows the release of oxygen from the red blood cells into the body.

If we breathe large volumes of air, we decrease the blood pH level, which doesn't help release the existing oxygen. Many think shortness of breath means a lack of oxygen. But the reality is that the existing oxygen isn't being released from the blood to the organs, as too much carbon dioxide is being expelled from our bodies by unregulated volumes of breath. We cannot hold our breath because we don't have carbon dioxide tolerance. *So, contrary to what you may think, when our breath rate is regulated and the volume of air is lowered, we feel more energetic!* Fatigue and excessive yawning are not always due to physical or mental exertion but could be the effect of suboptimal breathing.

Many breathing practices are advocated today, and the importance of having a routine that incorporates breath-work might not be new to many of us. *But our breathing efficiency is rooted in our lifestyle, which includes dietary choices, postural and movement habits. Without a change in these key elements, our breathing routines can have little or no effect.*

Segmental Breathing

This breathing is an effective method for beginners to bring down the volume of air we breathe per minute.

Level 1: Inhale from the nose in three instalments, with a mini pause between each segment. One inhalation is broken into three parts, so you are breathing in the same volume of air, but slowly, with a mini pause between each instalment. This naturally slows down the breath rate and reduces the volume of air you breathe, per minute.

The exhalation is in one go through the nose. If you are already out of breath with the inhalation and find it tough to exhale from the nose, then you can exhale from the mouth, as it is easier and brings instant peace and calm.

You may find breathing in three instalments tough. You can reduce it to two instalments to make it comfortable, as this breathing technique needs to be sustained continuously for 5–10 minutes. Getting out of breath is an indication you are pushing too much too quickly. Going slower is better. *Breathing efficiently is a lost art that needs to be cultivated through practice, just like playing a sport or musical instrument.*

Level 2: The next stage is to do the reverse, by taking in a regular inhalation and breaking down the exhalation into two or three instalments, through the nose or mouth.

Note: Never inhale from the mouth, only exhale.

Time how many breaths you can take per minute when you are practising level 1, and compare it with level 2. They should match. If there is a dissimilarity, it means you can't rush to level 3, as you need to work on equalizing your inhalation and exhalation capacity.

Level 3: For many, just the above two levels work like magic! Individuals who start with a normal breath rate of 25 breaths per minute easily achieve between 6–10 breaths per minute through practice. Those who find the first and second level easy can try the next level, which is breathing in as well as out in two or three instalments. This further reduces the volume we breathe to a mere 4 to 6 breaths per minute. This is a very achievable goal for many.

Retest: Always test your natural breath count before and after this exercise. It will give you insights into your progress.

Since our spontaneous breath rate tends to be higher when left unaware, if you are breathing only 4 or 6 breaths while practising, you will be able to achieve a regular breath rate lower than 10 breaths a minute. For the extremely enthusiastic, it does not end here, as the goal is to try breathing less than 10 breaths even during movement-based activities.

Why Are the Effects of Breathing Exercises and Meditation for Mental Health not Long-lasting?

Stress is a daily battle, and we cannot escape from it. Stress itself isn't the disease, but how we handle it or don't will determine its effects on our physiology. Those who have studied the Patanjali Yoga Sutras understand how breathing and mental health are closely interconnected. *The effects of most breathing techniques are short-lived and have partial benefits, because restrictions and shortcomings in the basic foundation of the body make the stress return.*

Nervous tension and stored emotions cause energy blocks in our connective tissue, which is made up of 70 per cent water.[33] Thus, our entire body, along with our muscles and soft tissue, is affected by our mental states. The problem is that most people counterbalance the mental tension with mental relaxation. But the body still holds on to those energy blocks that were created in our distressed states. It takes time and certain methods for the body to release the trauma caused by mental states. If the body is left unattended, these emotions surface as ailments or myofascial triggers. They can also surface in our dreams, creating sleep disturbances.[34]

Energy blocks are responsible for muscle tension that manifests subconsciously, as with tightness around the eyes, stiffness in the sole of the foot, tensing of the skull, clenching of the jaw or an elevated upper trapezius. Thus, our efforts to relax only our mental states aren't adequate for living at the peak of our well-being. The body is trapped with excess baggage, as it responds to the emotions that are still stored within it. *Thus, a parallel equivalence between our mental and physical body can be attained only through the release of our soft tissue.*

Below is a test to determine if you are deriving the maximum benefit from all your inputs for better mental health.

360-Degree Test for Optimal Breathing

Part 1: Lie down on your back and place your hand on your belly. With every inhalation, see if it expands, and with every exhalation, it should deflate like a balloon.

This is the most natural way to breathe while we are resting. For some, this rhythm is reversed, and they expand the belly with every exhalation and deflate it on every inhalation. In this case, the pattern needs to be relearnt and restored, as there is a shift in the breathing muscles utilized that compensate for the actual muscles. As babies, we did not need to learn to breathe. It was a natural ability. But normal breathing patterns get compromised with today's fast-paced life that alters diet, creates stress, worsens posture and contributes to ill health.

Part 2: This breathing pattern is what we use while we sit. Place a cushion under the sit-bones to elevate your back so you are not compressing the abdomen by slouching.

Place one hand on your chest and the other on the belly. Is the belly expanding with every inhalation and deflating with every exhalation? Some find the expansion of the belly impossible to do, as they naturally breathe more from the chest.

Notice the breathing pattern in the chest. Are you a heavy chest breather? Are your ribcage and shoulder elevated instead of expanding 360 degrees from the sides, back and chest? *If that is the case, then this breathing pattern makes your neck muscles and trapezius muscles get tighter with every breath.* This subtle action of breathing goes unnoticed by many. But as harmless as this may seem, it causes upper-back and neck pain. This breathing pattern is also seen when we are stressed and cannot breathe from the belly and are breathing heavily from the chest.

- When we sit, we spontaneously inhale passively and exhale actively, drawing the belly in towards the spine. This is a very gentle invisible action of the stabilizing muscles that maintains optimal posture. For many, this isn't natural. Toddlers, for example, sit perfectly well with straight backs. Their body does not restrict or alter their breath, and their breath helps stabilize their body.

Part 3: We will now try out the hollowing core technique in a seated position for this test. This test exposes myofascial restrictions in areas that can contribute to inefficient breathing.

- Take a deep breath in. The abdomen should expand like a balloon. On the exhalation (slowly from the mouth), shrink the abdomen from all sides.
- Retaining the shape and position of the spine, try to inhale and exhale, only from your ribcage and not the belly.
- On an inhalation, the ribcage should expand equally from all sides. To test this, place your hands on the sides of your ribcage. Feel the left and right sides of the ribcage expand laterally. If you feel only one side expanding, the other may be tight or inhibited.
- Place one hand on the chest and the other on the mid-back and inhale. Your belly should remain held in throughout the breathing process. Sometimes, some people have more movement in the chest compared to the back or vice versa.

It is imperative that the chest, back and the left and right sides of the ribcage expand equally and simultaneously with each breath. This indicates the standard of quality of a basic wholesome breath in an active position. *Restrictions in the chest, back or left or right side of the ribs will mean that other muscles are being used to breathe.* If each breath we take isn't a wholesome 360-degree breath, then how can we derive full mental benefit from our breathing and meditative techniques? How can the breath physically help stabilize the spine when the wrong muscles are being used for every breath?

We can get into all the breathing exercises the world offers, but if our torso lacks the capacity to expand, our breath rate will be high, making slow and deep breathing inefficacious. *You can practise regulated breathing and reap the benefits of a relaxed mind as well as controlled volumes of air. But their effects will last only for a short period, as your existing myofascial restrictions will increase your breath rate when your breath is left unchecked, inviting stress and anxiety back into your life. We can extend the benefit of our breathing and meditative practices by removing the myofascial restrictions that curtail it.*

To understand how myofascial restrictions curtail our breathing, let us distinguish between passive invisible breathing and perceptible visible breathing.

The intercostal muscle and diaphragm are the main muscles used in respiration. Along with them, the abdominal muscles—the inner and outer core—assist. The diaphragm is a dome-shaped muscle at the base of the lungs that separates the stomach cavity from the chest. It contracts on an inhalation and relaxes on an exhalation. When we are unaware, we are breathing passively. *The passive inhalations of an individual with superior breathing hardly display any visible movement in the chest. But the thoracic muscles still play a vital role in it.* There are eleven intercostal muscles between twelve ribs that help elevate the ribs during passive inhalation. They expand anteriorly, posteriorly as well as laterally when the thoracic cavity is enlarged, even though this might not be very visible to the eye. *When our passive inhalations become perceptible, then it is an indication of myofascial restriction.* Thus, besides the abdomen, all the other muscles surrounding the diaphragm as well as those muscles that assist the diaphragm in breathing need to be free of restrictions.

Addressing the Cause

Poor postural habits create tightness in the muscles in the trunk, which inhibits expansion of the breath. *This traps us in a loop of impaired breathing patterns that either lead to heavy chest breathing or rapid or shallow breaths that can contribute to an increase in psychological stress.* Daily stress, combined with faulty postures, increases myofascial restrictions, which makes every breath we take unwholesome. If the abdominals are taut due to faulty posture, or tight due to over-exercising, the diaphragm does not have the freedom to move downward as we inhale. It is constantly pushed upward and prevents deep breathing. It contributes to digestive issues, as it restricts movement of liquids and solid foods, as the oesophagus passes through the diaphragm into the stomach. Gut issues further usher in respiratory ailments.

Breathing in Relation to Weight Loss and Pathology

Diet: Our diet affects our oral health, respiration as well as sleep.[35] Globalization has impacted the food and nutrition systems of the world today.[36] An increase in the choice of food options has seen a proportional increase in respiratory disease and obesity. Today's culture exposes children and adults to fast foods that either use poor-quality oil, refined flour or are processed, packaged or frozen. A health study showed that Chinese Singaporeans who had a diet rich in meats, sodium and refined carbohydrates faced an increased risk of developing cough with phlegm, despite the apparent beneficial effects of their diet, which was high in fibre.[37] These dietary choices, including overindulgence in sugar, leads to excess mucus that blocks nasal passages, which causes mouth breathing and snoring.

Mouth breathing and blocked nasal passages affect sleep and, over a period of time, lead to deformed jawlines and dental problems. If you are more susceptible to dental issues, check your diet, nasal passages and breathing patterns throughout the day and night. Mouth breathing and snoring lead to dehydration,[38] which has other effects on the entire physiology. Mouth breathing or blocked nasal passages also lead to excessive yawning during the day or while exercising. It is a signal from the body that it lacks the efficient transportation of oxygen to various body parts.

Eating heavy fried foods and consuming excess sugar and alcohol increase obesity, which affects our breathing during sleep. The quality of our sleep is more important than the number of hours we sleep. Blocked nasal passages lead to disturbed sleep. This increases restlessness and anxiety and decreases brain functions, like concentration and memory. Sleep disorders like sleep apnoea are on the rise, and 22 per cent Indians, including children, suffer from snoring.[39]

Overeating: You simply cannot control the volume of air you breathe if you are an overeater. The combination of rapid breathing and overeating creates stress on the pancreas as we intensify the load on the digestive system. The final outcome is pre-diabetes,[40] where health is further compromised. Overeating at even one meal can lead to heaviness in breathing.

Hard-to-digest foods can have the same impact as overeating, because they lead to rapid breathing. These foods can be of any kind. For some people, it is oily food or dairy, and for some it could be meat or wheat. The more you train your belly to consume smaller quantities of food, the less you will be able to overeat.

Weight loss: Do you eat healthy but can't seem to keep your weight down? Have you been to all the nutritionists in the city, yet their diet programmes and exercise just don't seem to have the desired effect? An easy, simple solution would be to check your breathing.

How much air we breathe has a direct impact on our metabolism, as it regulates appetite and reduces hunger cravings without the need to suppress it. The stomach shrinks, hunger is curbed as our overall physiology improves. Lower volumes of air retain the carbon dioxide in the body, thereby increasing the oxygen flow to the pancreas, which then processes foods more efficiently. Scientific research has proved that breath-reduction exercises, sustained over a period of time, decrease the waist–hip ratio.[41] As Patrick McKeown writes, 'For every 5 kgs of fat loss in our bodies 80 percent of it comes out through the lungs as carbon dioxide mixed with a bit of water vapour, the rest being sweat or urine. Losing weight is as easy as breathing as the lungs are the weight regulating system of the body.'[42]

Kapaalbati and *bastrika* have been promoted as the leading weight loss breathing exercises. These breathing exercises that involve hyperventilation are practised by a large section of the Indian population and have their benefits in clearing the mucus and unblocking nasal passages. *But if we want better balance in our physiology, then there must also be an awareness to reduce the volumes of air we breathe.* To quote Patrick McKeown again, 'Breathing the right volume of air throughout the day keeps burning calories even in passive activities like sitting and sleeping thus increasing the body's efficiency and metabolism.'[43]

Periodic checks on how we are breathing should be made throughout the day. We always have ideal moments like when watching Netflix, travelling or showering, so we all have plenty of time to practise breath regulation. It is the easiest way you can de-stress and enjoy a meditative experience, which comes with dual health benefits.

Pathology: Faulty diets and eating habits accompanied with stress and anxiety mess up our pathology. Regulated breathing is the cheapest, most natural and effortless mechanism our body is equipped with to neutralize the effects of stress. I haven't met anyone with regulated and controlled breathing habits who suffers from the ill-effects of stress, such as a messed-up pathology and obesity. We cannot separate health from breath, or our breath from pathology, as the way we breathe affects the functioning of the entire body.

4

What Is My Relationship with Pain?

Chronic pain is not all about the body, and it is not all about the brain—it is everything. Target everything! Take back your life.—Dr Sean Mackey

What do we think about pain? For some, it is an inconvenience while others fear or simply ignore it. None of these approaches serve us. We need to reassess our relationship with pain so we can use it as a warning signal rather than treat it as a hindrance, nuisance or threat.

Balms and painkillers were invented so we could cover up the pain while masking the actual problem and move on with life. But pain isn't the problem—it is only a symptom. The actual problem lies elsewhere but we kill the messenger by using painkillers and balms, before we get the message. Sure, they help when pain is overpowering our lives, but the actual dysfunction and inflammation existed in the body long before the pain surfaced. So, *ignoring pain and covering it up doesn't demonstrate a healthy relationship with pain, as it is inimical to our well-being.*

Life is busy and completing our daily tasks is important. But the message that pain gives us is equally important. We embrace all other warning signs and are up-to-date with upgrading and updating our computers, phones and apps. *How about using the warning sign of pain as an indication to update and upgrade ourselves?*

With our sedentary life, the working of the body is compromised since we perform only impaired movements. The intelligent body allows compensatory movements because of our mobility restrictions. *Compensatory patterns can exist with or without pain.* The body was designed to adapt easily and will adopt a poor movement pattern so it can survive. This eventually leads to dysfunction in other body parts, so it is necessary to troubleshoot and correct even the smallest discomfort and pain.

Some consider pain an unpleasant feeling and sometimes fear the worst-case scenario—internal damage. This is often a misconception, as pain is complex and can't always be directly related to physical causes. Our body is also affected by emotions, muscle soreness or muscle triggers. The role of pain is to alert us and protect a body part or parts that the brain *thinks* are damaged. The brain can be right or wrong.[1] *Therefore, it is crucial to understand that pain originates from the brain and not from a body part.*[2] Reassessing pain is important, as it can put a halt to many activities. *Pain can exist even in the absence of tissue damage because it results from the perception of a threat and perceptions are not always reality.* Pain can just be a signal with no major internal danger or damage. We shouldn't confuse the threat of pain with an actual injury.

Here are some reasons pain can occur without internal damage:

Psychological Pain

Most of us are aware and might have even experienced how mental stress can cause physical symptoms. Negative emotions, thoughts, perceptions and stress increase adrenaline and cortisol that keep the body in fight-or-flight mode, as it constantly sees a red flag indicating danger. Psychological pain and emotions can contribute to or worsen physical pain, such as headaches and muscular pains that already exist in the body. Stomach disorders or ache, sleep disorders, dizziness, nausea and anxiety are other kinds of pain that can arise due to lack of mental and emotional health. Increased heart rate and blood pressure, poor immunity, psoriasis, autoimmune diseases and rheumatic arthritis are some other effects of stress and anxiety.

When some doctors don't have solutions to a patient's problems, they attribute the issue to the patient's mental attitude, don't take the pain seriously and show such patients the door. There are also some individuals who don't agree with the view that there is a connection between mental and physical health. Yet those who believe it don't know the connection that could be the probable cause of pain in their own bodies. As unreal as psychosomatic problems may seem, their symptoms are very real, and the distress from these symptoms often lasts a lifetime for those who don't resolve their emotional issues. As Michael J. Shea writes, 'Research proves that loneliness, depression, hope and fear and the pain of dealing with pain are very valid psychological reasons for myofascial pain which resurfaces even after treatment.'[3]

Delayedd Onset Muscle Soreness (DOMS)

Many people have a tough time distinguishing DOMS from pain that could be an actual risk or threat.[4] DOMS occurs 12–48 hours after a workout and can last for one day or even one and a half weeks. Many individuals don't even like the feeling of their muscles overworking during exercise and refuse to push past a threshold.

The pain from DOMS isn't actual pain but soreness caused when there is a disruption of the muscle fibrils. When we push ourselves harder than usual or use newer muscle groups that have never been worked out, or simply start an exercise routine after a long period of inactivity, DOMS sets in. A muscle strain will cause immediate pain that is concentrated in a small area. This is what differentiates muscle strain from DOMS, as DOMS usually involves many muscle groups and larger areas of discomfort.

DOMS shouldn't be treated as a threat to our comfort, nor should one get too anxious about damaged tissue. No treatment is required for DOMS, as it usually resolves itself within a week. To reduce the discomfort, having a scoop of L-Glutamine,[5] foam-rolling the sore area and icing can help.

Muscle Triggers

Muscle triggers or micro-cramps are an example of the confusion the brain creates when it misconceives a pain signal and perceives it as a risk/actual threat.[6] The various reasons that contribute towards muscle triggers in the body are discussed below.

Myofascial pain syndrome is when chronic pain is experienced because of too many trigger points. These should be considered more as 'irritants' that need attention rather than major 'threats'. The nastier the trigger point, the more the pain, but there may be exceptions.

When triggers are dissolved by a therapist or masseur, it feels like a miracle! But in truth, triggers are the most prevalent form of physical aches and pains concurrent with today's lifestyle. This book shares easy methods to resolve your aches and pains, which you can do by yourself anywhere, anytime. You will never feel helpless with pain and immobility while travelling or get stuck in a situation with no external support. Regular release of our tissues makes it healthy and prevents us from getting into situations where pain gets intolerable.

Intense pain is sometimes misleading. This isn't a point that should lead you to neglect troubleshooting the pain area. Pain is a messenger, informing us that something needs attention. It is better to act on the message—understand what kind of pain it is and what could be its probable causes. It is not correct or wise to suppress the signals themselves with painkillers (unless the pain is unbearable). Pain is the only method of communication that the brain has to indicate whether the body has fully recovered or not.

Three golden rules apply when it comes to pain:

1. Don't be your own doctor or therapist by jumping to conclusions. Always seek advice from a professional.
2. Don't neglect pain if it persists beyond a week.
3. Don't panic—it is most likely nothing.

An individual's life experiences mould their concept of pain and its effects, so it is essential to re-evaluate our beliefs about pain. The International Association for the Study of Pain (IASP) has proposed a new definition of pain—'An aversive sensory and emotional experience, typically caused by, or resembling that which is caused by, an actual or potential tissue injury'.[7] Thus, it is clear that pain is a sensation that is very individualistic, depending on the psychological and physiological intelligence of each individual.

5

Most Common Reasons for Pain

The most underrated component of health is tissue health. Protecting our joints comes by maintaining the quality of the tissue that slides and glides over them. If it is taut, lumpy and bumpy, it affects the joints and limits the range of motion. This creates an unnecessary load, which eventually wears out the joints. The aches and pains we deal with are a cumulative result of the stress our tissues undergo because of the various factors touched upon below:

Stored Emotions and Muscle Tension

Stress, anxiety and stored negative thoughts and emotions create imbalance in the autonomic nervous system that is responsible for regulating the heart rate, blood pressure, breathing and digestion. The effect is a weakened immune system highly susceptible to disease. Unresolved mental issues and stored emotions surface in our dreams at night, create mental stress while we sleep and can manifest in a shoulder or neck pain upon waking up. Grinding our teeth, tightening the jaw and clenching and cracking the fingers and toes, fidgeting, shaking a leg and tapping the heel are all indications of emotional stress. Research today suggests that most of our health problems are psychosomatic.[1] Our entire body, along with our muscles and soft tissue, is affected by nervous tension. Most individuals will tackle their ailments by visiting the doctor, who will prescribe some medication to balance heart rate, high blood pressure, anxiety and gut-related issues. But if we were to take a step back, then de-stressing the autonomic nervous system is the cure.

Everyone has a stress buster today, but the popular relaxation choices are smoking, drinking, drugs and mental distractions like watching movies and TV series non-stop, binge eating and partying. These might make us feel temporarily relaxed, but anxiety and stress return the next day. None of these choices counterbalance the muscular tensions and stress stored in our soft tissue. Some may opt for healthier choices, like participating in physical endurance challenges to channel their emotions and thoughts, while others feel great with hobbies like a sport, but all of these mediums actually leave our tissues with more stress and strain.

The therapeutic use of the *right* relaxation techniques for the mind and body respectively, is the only way we can ward off the effects of daily muscular and nervous tension. Mental stress requires mental relaxation. Muscle tension can be countered with the release techniques shared below. They offer a solution that loosens up our muscles and immediately induces relaxation. These release techniques can benefit us mentally and physically, as they soothe our muscle and tissue, which automatically takes the edge off mental tension.

Insufficient Hydration

Hydration is vital to preserving the quality of our tissue and regulating our breathing and is crucial for the efficient functioning of all our organs. The body is made up of two-thirds water, so our hydration levels affect everything.

The fascia, which is the connective tissue found under the skin, runs through the whole body. This dissectible tissue stabilizes, imparts strength, separates muscles and attaches and encloses organs. Our bones, nerves and blood vessels are held together because of connective tissue, which is made of 70 per cent water! Proteoglycans hold water in our fascial system to keep it supple. So, we can imagine the effect even slight dehydration can have on the entire body.

People experience cramping in their stretches suddenly after a summer break, wondering why so much stiffness has suddenly set in. These are simply symptoms of dehydration that have gone unnoticed. If you are one of those who have a lot of knotty tissue, then a hydration diet that improves its quality should be part of the healing process, along with self-myofascial release.

Most people don't drink enough water. Even those who do, don't know how to such that it is absorbed by the cells and keeps them nourished. Even if we are drinking the required three litres a day, we can still be dehydrated. If you are waiting to feel thirsty and then sip water, you are already dehydrated. This is because by the time the brain gives the signal that you are thirsty, your body is already dried out.

The right way to hydrate is to sip not more than 150 ml water every ten minutes. The usual tendency for most is to wait till one is thirsty and then chug down a glass of water. But by drinking water in this manner all of it isn't absorbed by the cells. The proof of it is seen in prolonged urination. The need to urinate more than six to seven times a day is also a sign of over hydration, where water is simply flushed out of the system without getting absorbed.

Even if we are slightly dehydrated, the body can lose power and energy to function at its peak.[2] If you think you are functioning at the peak of your ability, think again, as research has proven that dehydration affects mood, attention, memory and motor coordination.[3] I always think of water as nourishment for the brain and its functions. Sitting in air-conditioning[4] all day with UV lights,[5] little exposure to natural light or too much exposure to the sun, staring into computer screens, tablets and phones—all this is part of the process of dehydration on a daily basis. Simply chugging down three litres of water isn't enough to counteract these effects. The indirect effect of dehydration is seen in the tightness and stiffness in tissue that causes aches and pains.

Vitamin Deficiencies

For some individuals, a regular tissue maintenance programme may not be enough to combat aches and pains if there is an underlying deficiency or hormonal or muscular imbalance. Research has proven that subclinical hypothyroidism, iron insufficiency, Vitamin B and D and magnesium insufficiency, estrogen and testosterone deficiency and the use of statins can interfere with pain patterns in the body.[6] It is necessary to address these factors internally before embarking on your journey to becoming pain-free.

Many consider lack of vitamin D3 and B12 as new-age propaganda. But an immediate increase in these levels has a magical effect on aches and pains. In order to preserve and maintain our tissue health, constantly monitoring these levels at any age is vital. Individuals stuck with hormonal issues like hypothyroidism benefit largely from the myofascial self-care programme. It reduces the intensity and regularity of cramps and pains that become an inconvenience, as they occur at any time, even in the middle of the night. For those who are on statins and prefer to choose the easy path of managing blood panels with a fifteen-second solution need to rethink their choice, as this comes with its own side-effects namely, muscle pain and damage, liver damage, onset of type 2 diabetes and neurological side effects.[7]

Movement Dysfunction and Imbalanced Approach Towards the Exposure of Load

Damage to our soft tissue can occur through injury, undergoing surgery and being left with scar tissue, underuse or overuse of muscles and postural stress. Standing for long hours can strain the lower limbs, feet and tender spots in the back. Sharp points of pain can develop along the spine if you lift a heavy object that you are not used to. Static balance is impaired in the forward head posture, which creates an imbalanced load and leads to a more widespread effect on the entire body.[8] Even after an asthmatic attack or respiratory infection, the chest and intercostal muscles tighten as you cough. Suddenly taking up fitness activities after a long break can cause muscle strains and sprains, leaving tender tight spots and trigger points in surrounding areas in the tissue. The slight discomfort we experience after wearing high heels or tight shoes can also restrict the tissue in our feet. Inappropriately designed workspaces and prolonged use of keyboards for typing can precipitate neck, shoulder and wrist pain.

Why Is Soft-Tissue Maintenance Essential?

Triggers that develop can be lumpy knots the size of a golf ball or they can be micro-contractions that have the ability to produce immense pain, even if they are as tiny as a grain of sand. They are a nuisance and can be linked to several problems such as headaches, migraines, blurred vision, dizziness, a painful spot or referred pain, stiff and painful joints, and tight musculature that decreases efficiency by reducing strength.

Referred pain* is experienced by many as a result of today's lifestyle.

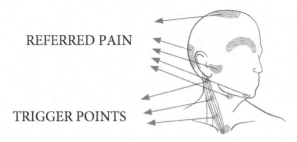

REFERRED PAIN

TRIGGER POINTS

---

* Referred pain is when you feel pain in one part of your body but it is actually stemming from another part of your body.

This is how a trigger point in one area can produce referred pain or a different symptom in another area. *Imbalanced tissue health can lead to innumerable issues that might have no diagnosis but are still experienced as being life-threatening. Many individuals are in the dark about how daily soft-tissue release can improve their quality of life and address the issues that are misdiagnosed or undetected.*

As we age, the quality of our tissue determines how far we can push and endure strenuous movements, and move or not move without getting stiff or developing trigger points. To quickly recover and rebuild tissue at any age, it is essential we adhere to the various aspects mentioned above that enhance our tissue health. If you are determined to augment tissue health, then a regimen that improves flexibility and mobility is the answer.

6

Soft-Tissue Release to Fix Common Aches and Pains

The release techniques shared in this section form an independent maintenance solution to counterbalance and troubleshoot the repetitive stress and pain endured on a daily basis in our jobs, hobbies and activities.

Besides good hydration and adequate vitamin intake, soft-tissue release is the key to release emotional, mental and physical stress. Our foundational movement skills reduce the impact of repetitive stress in our daily life. When accompanied by these soft-tissue releases, the quality of our tissue and mobility increase considerably. Even if we don't suffer from any aches and pains, regular use of these techniques makes us get away with any kind of postural stress our environment may impose on us. The fewer the constraints, the more wholesome our movements become. This is where this self-care maintenance routine must be a ritual. With learning to 'move right', the need for daily maintenance also decreases with time, as bodies are not exposed to stress and strain.

When Do We Perform Soft-Tissue Release?

These can be performed in a home or desk-bound environment, at the gym, while travelling or as pre- or post-care during fitness activities. Since this self-massage eases the mind and body and induces relaxation, those who have trouble sleeping can benefit if they perform it before bedtime. Those niggling aches and pains are easily taken care of with the techniques prescribed. However, care should be taken not to further damage tissue that is already injured. Performing some of these releases before a yoga class can make stretching even more enjoyable.

- While treating painful areas be gentle with yourself. Begin by applying less pressure, then slowly increase it to the extent you can tolerate. Usually, a pain of five on a scale of ten is considered appropriate. If you are too gentle, you won't get results, and if you exert too much pressure too quickly, bruising may occur. Individuals who are on blood thinners and corticosteroids are more susceptible to bruising and should be careful. Initially, work less but work more often—every day or every alternate day, depending on how sore the area is. You can ice the areas worked on if you feel they have become too tender after release. The beauty of this method is that you are the master and judge of your own pain. So, applying the right amount of pressure is in your hands. Soft-tissue release is safe to implement every day, especially if you are trying to troubleshoot different areas of tightness each day.

- Always work around the problem areas upwards, downwards, towards the left and right sides. Remember, you are treating a band of tissue, even if you experience pain on just a particular spot. The surrounding tissue also gets affected, since everything is connected.

- It isn't wise to perform soft-tissue release right before exercise. It is usually preferred after exercise, since relaxing your muscles right before a workout may make them lose their ability to contract. However, there are certain specific times where you may have to fix a particular troublesome area if it is preventing you from performing your exercise or activity with ease. Soft-tissue release can be performed on the go anywhere, while you are commuting or sitting in the office, or at any time, even for a few minutes to half an hour. It can be performed multiple times a day on different body parts and can be used to induce relaxation and ease out common symptoms.

General massages are good to flush out tissue and increase circulation. However, if you need to troubleshoot certain sticky spots that need more attention, then the application of the tools and techniques prescribed can help you go very deep into the layers of connective tissue. The techniques shared below eliminate any soft-tissue restrictions by breaking up myofascial adhesions and trigger points that generate other symptoms. Easing out ailments like headaches, chest pains, pelvic floor dysfunction, respiratory issues and others mentioned earlier requires an understanding of the possible areas that can cause these symptoms. This is where general massages have their limitations.

Tools Used for Soft-Tissue Release

Soft-tissue release is something that can be done anytime, anywhere, using any tool. Any solid surface that digs into our musculature can be used to ease soreness, pain or tightness. Common household items like a pen, rolling pin, aluminium or curtain rod, a cooking aid like a firm silicon and wooden spatula can be used for effective release. The most commonly used tool that works for most of the body parts are balls of different sizes and varieties.

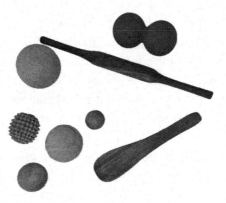

Crazy balls, tennis ball, squash ball, rolling pin,
peanut ball, wooden spatula

You might want to start with objects you already have at home and then invest in some of these as you get better at it. Once you get a hang of these techniques, you can be innovative and use any object to give yourself a little massage on the go. At your office desk, you may want to use the rounded, blunt end of your pen to dig into your forearm or palm. If I'm sitting on a chair, I may use its edge to dig into my upper back, or I may use the edge of a bed to release my hamstrings.

Stretching after Soft-Tissue Release

Whenever one is trying to achieve length in a muscle, releasing trigger points or taut bands of tissue is essential before stretching. However, simply performing the release and not stretching areas of tissue may not result in the desired effect. Dynamic stretching is always preferred before a static stretch, as it opens up joints and allows relaxation while performing the static stretch.

There are many techniques when it comes to stretching, but stretching must be experienced as a sense of ease in the body and mind. Anything that is forced and painful will not lengthen the muscle but will create further tightness and hotspots. If a stretch feels stuck and painful, then it needs more soft-tissue release. You may also try to find other areas that may be contributing to the tightness in the region. For some individuals who are very tight, it may take a few days of releasing to achieve the desired range of motion. A key element is the breath while stretching. You have to breathe in order to relax and go deeper so the muscle can lengthen.

Head, Neck and Jaw

- **Pain symptoms experienced**
  Head, neck and jaw triggers may lead to symptoms like dizziness, blurred vision,[1] visual disturbances, vertigo,[2] [3]

tinnitus (ringing in the ears),[4] hearing problems, temporomandibular joint (TMJ) dysfunction,[5] migraine,[6] headaches, nausea,[7] face pain,[8] imbalance, back of head/ neck pain, pain on the side of the neck.

- **Why and how this soft-tissue release can help you**
  Improvements and changes can be seen in the forward head posture, provided the poor habits that lead to stress and degeneration are taken care of. For individuals in professions that require looking down constantly, or if you tend to use digital devices all day, you will find a sense of ease. Even children and adults who don't suffer any aches and pains can perform this routine as a daily maintenance to prevent degenerative changes in the neck. Individuals who grit their teeth at night or have frequent headaches, migraines or ringing in the ears must give this routine a chance to see if there are any trigger points that are sending out pain signals.

  A lot of conditions can be misdiagnosed if the underlying problem is unidentified myofascial triggers. When I suffered imbalance and unsteadiness in the head, even after a battery of all the possible tests, MRIs and pointless visits to the ENT, orthopaedic, neurologist, general physician and even the dentist, there was no medical correlation. I was finally free of my symptoms after soft-tissue release of the neck, head and jaw. This section has helped many individuals to get rid of sudden migraines, vertigos and other traumatizing effects of cervical ailments.

- **Affected areas**

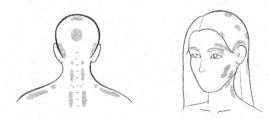

Use this guide to check if these are the same areas of pain/symptoms that you suffer. It is crucial to note that if you are targeting only the pain areas and ignoring the surrounding areas, your pain is likely to return or may decrease only partially. Our body is an endless myofascial web where everything is connected, therefore working the surrounding areas ensures an ease in the whole structure. For those who would like to go a step further, it is wise to try the techniques of the shoulder, upper back and mid-back to gain permanent results, since our posture and movements involve a lot of muscles.

Some individuals may also find their symptoms overlapping in two areas, such as the neck and shoulder. Some may have issues in three. I have met a 24-year-old who had symptoms starting from the neck, shoulder, lower back, mid-back, knee, right down to the ankle! Your gut can trigger neck pain, headaches and migraines. Your elbow, forearm and chest can also contribute to neck pain. Thus performing self-myofascial release everyday on the whole body, one body part at a time, is ideal. Exploring various areas, to see what eases your pain, is the self-education that will enlighten you to the areas that are more susceptible to developing hotspots for you.

- **Tools**
  - o Ball: investments in balls of various sizes and softness will give you a better understanding of how each area can be treated. Crazy balls, squash balls and tennis balls can be used to treat delicate areas and tender hotspots since they are softer. Harder balls like yoga balls, lacrosse balls and golf balls can be used for areas that can take more pressure as you can go deeper with them. If you are treating an area every day for a few days, then you may feel like choosing a harder tool on the second day, to go deeper into the release as your tissue opens up.
  - o Fingers: Use your fingers for areas that feel too painful, but try to save them for areas of the neck and other tender portions of the body where it is dangerous to use an external tool. Using your fingers first over a painful area is a good way to examine what areas feel tighter and more painful than the others.

- **Soft-tissue release techniques**
  Neck—Sternocleidomastoid

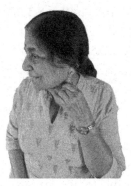

This area is best treated with fingers. Turn your head to one side to locate the sternocleidomastoid. Run your fingers along the thick band of muscle, gently but firmly, trying to ease out lumpy or taut areas along the entire length of the muscle. If a particular spot feels tender or sends radiating pain in any direction away from the spot you are treating, then apply a constant pressure that you can endure till the radiating pain subsides. You will also experience that the intensity of pain reduces in non-radiating spots as you press on them for a while. You can then move on to the next spot in the same muscle, once you feel some degree of ease has set in.

The amount of time required for each muscle and each hotspot depends on various factors like the quality of your tissue, how taut or tight it is and how many areas feel painful. Be patient, have faith and try to connect with your body through the process. To gain confidence and competence in self-myofascial release, it is always wiser to attend a course* to learn the finer nuances in a practical setting to achieve the best results.

Posterior Neck Muscles

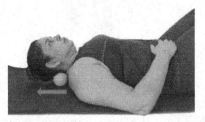

Easing out the posterior neck is non-negotiable for most individuals. Bending the neck forward to look at the phone

---

* See www.movebetterwellness.in.

screen, wristwatch, computer or devices is a habit most find difficult to change. Take a medium to hard ball and lie on your back on a hard surface, while you slowly move the ball over one side of the posterior neck. Make sure you are travelling parallel to the discs of the neck and not in the centre, over the bone. Roll the ball up and down and pause at tight or painful spots till they ease out. Then roll over the whole area to smoothen out the surface.

Upper, Middle and Lower Trapezius

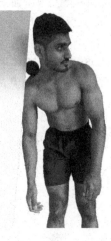

Locate the lumpy areas of the *upper trapezius*. Take a hard ball and place it on the muscle. Then go towards the edge of a wall and push the ball into the muscle with your arm dangling. Support the ball with the other hand and move it left, right, up and down till the upper trapezius feels significantly soft and smooth.

After using the ball to clear the topmost superficial surface, you can use your fingers to pinch the front and back of the upper trapezius to ease out the sides.

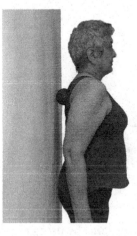

Use a medium to soft ball and lean against a wall and move upward, downward, right and left on both sides of the *middle trapezius* along the whole band of muscle.

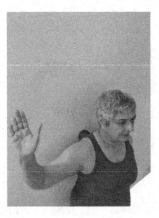

You can rotate your arm upwards and sideways while holding the ball on a hotspot. Alternatively, you can choose to lie down on the floor with the ball for this release.

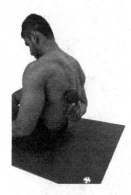

Ease out the *lower trapezius* by using a hard ball between you and a wall or the floor. Ensure you move left, right, up and down around the whole area.

Head—Temporalis

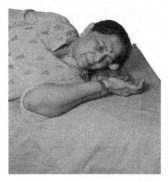

Lie down on your side. Ensure the shoulder has enough space and isn't in the way. For this purpose, I like to use a yoga block or a hardbound book that is readily available in every house. Place the ball on the block and lay your head on the temporalis muscle. Stay with each hotspot till it eases out. This may take time, but the post-release feeling is liberating.

Move in circles or diagonally from the sides upwards to smoothen out the surface.

Warning: Be careful of hair being pulled during this release.

Suboccipitals

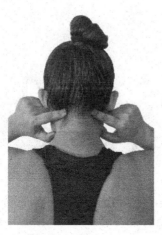

If you feel the back of your head with your fingers, you will find two points on the sides of the base of the head that depress. You want to take a medium to hard ball into this depression and lie down till these tender spots feel less torturesome.

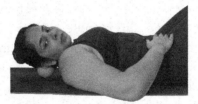

Then move upwards and target the points above each side. Stay with them while moving the head slightly right and left to dig deeper and ease out these regions.

Jaw—Masseter

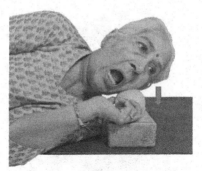

Take a medium-to-hard massage ball and place it around the masseter muscle as you lie on your side. Apply gentle pressure downward into the ball with your head. Try seeking painful spots in the surrounding areas and apply a constant pressure for thirty seconds on the points that hurt. Then open the mouth wide and close it multiple times to mobilize it after the pain slightly subsides.

- **Stretches**

  Myofascial release is incomplete without stretches that lengthen the tissue.

Neck

Stretch 1

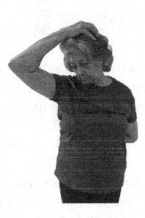

Place the arm of the side you want to stretch behind your back, as shown in the image above. This can be skipped if your arm doesn't have the ability to turn back. Start by turning the neck towards the opposite side of the arm. Hold your head with your hand and pull it down. Hold for thirty seconds or more. Overstretching the neck can make it taut. The next step of the stretch is to slowly shift the gaze and look down for thirty seconds. This step can be done dynamically as well as passively.

Stretch 2

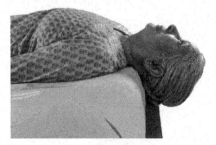

Those who have fatigue or pain at the back of the neck benefit from this simple stretch after the posterior neck release. Performing this stretch after a long day's work gives relief. Simply lie down on the edge of the bed and throw your head back for 2–3 minutes. The head must be supported and not dangle.

Those with pinched nerves must avoid any of the neck stretches and releases and must perform exercises only with the guidance of their physiotherapist.

Trapezius

Put your body weight on the arms in the quadruped position. Perform full range shoulder circles. This is a dynamic exercise used to determine if the shoulder blades are moving freely in an upward, downward, protracted and retracted motion. If you feel any constriction or pain at any angle, then massage of the upper, middle and lower trapezius is needed. You can also refer to the techniques of the upper back.

Jaw

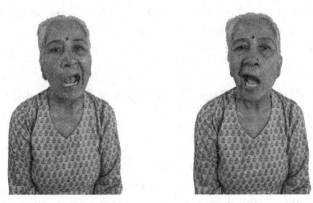

Open the jaw wide in length and breadth. Then mobilize it by moving it left and right. Perform this stretch multiple times a day for thirty seconds.

Eye Exercises

These exercises also come handy if you have any issues related to the neck and head. Our myofascial restrictions can cause an imbalance in our vision and vice versa. We are constantly staring at screens close to the face, which creates changes not only in our vision and also in our balance and posture. Yoga will have you do your eye exercises in the morning, but I would prescribe a minute of these in the middle of your day or towards the end, to counter all the stress the eyes have undergone through the day. I find these refreshing to the eyes if performed every few hours, especially if your work involves staring at a computer screen constantly.

Place the thumb in front between the eyes. Stare at the tip of the thumb and move the thumb backwards and forwards a few times. Then make a figure eight (8) clockwise and anticlockwise a few times.

Shoulder, Upper Back, Mid-back and Upper Limbs

Pain symptoms experienced:

- Shoulder pains in the anterior, posterior or middle of the shoulder, shoulder impingements, reduced range of motion in the shoulders and frozen shoulders.
- Pain in the upper back and mid-back due to long hours of postural stress.
- Pain experienced in the upper limbs, during and after sleep.
- Chest pains, false cardiac arrhythmia, angina symptoms[9] and heartburn are other symptoms due to myofascial triggers in these areas.
- Respiratory issues, breathing inefficiency and restrictions, indigestion and pelvic floor dysfunction.[10]
- Anxiety and depression[11] are the other symptoms that can surface as a result of unhealthy tissue in this region.

Why and how this soft-tissue release can help you

Rounded shoulders and hunched backs are improved with soft-tissue release, and their corresponding pain symptoms disappear.

The pain caused by gas which is trapped in the mid-back or chest due to an increase in stomach acids is greatly reduced with use of this section.

Hunched backs and rounded shoulders have an impact on our breathing, digestion, pelvic floor, cardiac functions and the efficient functioning of the brain. All these symptoms are eased out and improve after soft-tissue release.

If you are one of those who can feel a lot of clicks and hear grinding noises from the shoulder and upper back region, then a soft-tissue release on these surfaces should be a priority in order to prevent any future damage and deterioration of the joint.

Even if you are pain-free and desire to improve shoulder mobility, ease out the muscles of the upper back and increase performance on the side that you opt to play your single-hand sport. Regular release of these areas is a must for those keen individuals.

The abuse of a single preferred arm occurs while carrying a heavy bag daily on only one shoulder or using the computer, painting, photography and other hobbies. Regular myofascial release helps take care of the abuse and strain that results from this overuse.

Those who struggle to get relief from shoulder impingements need to take corrective measures to reduce internally rotated shoulders by strengthening the postural muscles. This ensures the shoulder is automatically repositioned and kept in its place through the day, improving impingement issues eventually. The upper back is intrinsically connected to the neck and vice versa, so if you are dealing with neck and head issues, these techniques used in combination will heighten the ease you feel in the entire torso.

Sherene, 60 years old, from Canada had a frozen shoulder which began functioning normally within five months of using these techniques. The speed of recovery from shoulder pathologies is dramatic when used alongside the conventional treatment methods.

- **Affected areas**

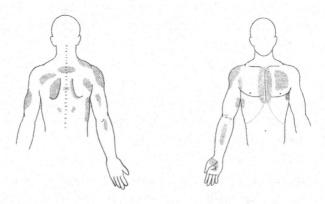

Check to see if these areas represent your pain areas. Sometimes you may need to work with techniques of the neck as well as the elbow and forearm muscles to get complete relief. Muscles of the rotator cuff are responsible for the majority of the pains and restrictions of the shoulder, but one must not undermine the trigger points in the muscles of the neck, the spinal muscles (latissimus dorsi) and upper arm, which can also be an underlying cause of pain and loss of mobility in the upper-back region. So if you're trying out these soft-tissue releases for the first time then, releasing all of these areas is imperative.

- **Tools**

    Medium-to-hard balls are best for these areas. Try soft-tissue release with a variety of different sized balls and hardness to see what gives you the maximum relief in each area.

- **Soft-tissue release techniques**

    Posterior rotator cuff muscles:

    The supraspinatus, infraspinatus and teres minor are the muscles released to ease rotator cuff issues. These generally tend to be tender and painful even if you don't have any shoulder issues. While performing the soft-tissue release on these areas, you may experience a 'pins and needles' kind of sensation. Don't panic; just breathe into it till you find the tissue easing out.

Supraspinatus

If you have trouble bringing the arm behind, this release is for you.

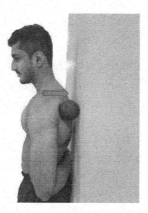

Try and bring the arm behind as much as you can (those who are completely stuck can avoid this movement). Dig a hard ball into the wall and push into the *supraspinatus*. Hold and breathe into the pain until comfortable. After a few breaths, try to go deeper in the stretch as you release. Getting back this range of motion is a gradual process.

Infraspinatus

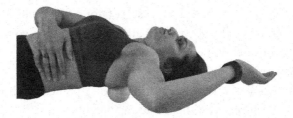

Lie down on your back and place a medium/hard ball on the shoulder blade surfaces.

Try to stretch the arm as the ball penetrates different areas of each surface.

Teres minor

You may accidentally dig into the teres minor muscle while trying to ease out the infraspinatus. This is a small but painful area for most individuals who have poor upper-back posture and strength.

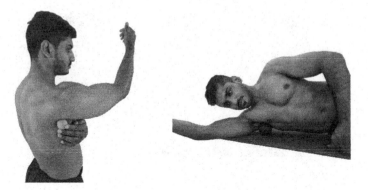

Place a medium/hard ball on the teres minor while lying down. To locate this area, find a tender spot next to the posterior side of the armpit. Locate the area first with your fingers. Use a smaller hard ball to dig into the area easily. Bring your arm out overhead and tilt slightly to the side, rolling the ball forward towards the armpit. Go back and forth, up and down in micro-movements. Don't worry if there is extreme pain in this region. Breathe into it.

Posterior deltoid pain, middle deltoid pain and anterior shoulder pain

The rotator cuff releases may need to be followed up with deltoid releases to give the finishing touches to alleviate your shoulder pain and increase mobility.

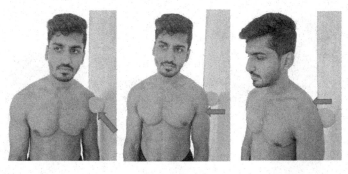

Anterior   Middle   Posterior

This release can be performed lying down or while standing against a wall. Use a medium/hard ball. As shown in the illustration, locate the posterior, middle as well as anterior parts of the deltoid and push the ball into these areas one spot at a time. Breathe into the areas that feel tender, tight or taut.

The shoulder and upper-back region are incomplete without the soft-tissue release of the rhomboid, latissimus dorsi and chest. Massage of these regions assist in better breathing and feeling of lightness in the upper-back region. These areas help alleviate stress and anxiety and promote a post-relaxation feeling in the mind and body.

Latissimus Dorsi

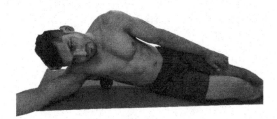

Take a hard ball to target the area under the shoulder blades. Lie down on the back on the floor or stand against a wall and breathe into hotspots (triggers) you may find in this region. Intuitively work in circular movements or upward and downward strokes.

The latissimus dorsi is a large muscle that extends to the sides of the torso. For this area, use a medium/hard ball while lying on the side with the arm extended overhead. You can increase or decrease the pressure by lowering or supporting the head.

Chest Muscles

Rounded shoulders and hunchback postures keep the chest muscles in a contracted state, which prevents wholesome and efficient breathing. Anxiety, depression and palpitations and apparent heart attacks are the effects of myofascial restrictions in these areas. There is a difference between pains of cardiac origin and those arising from the chest wall.[12] Besides these alarming symptoms, the chest muscles can contribute to shoulder, breast and forearm pains, accompanied with numbness and tingling sensations in the arm and palm. Tightness of the chest muscles can interfere with surgical procedures as well as post-surgical recovery, creating false symptoms of aches or uneasiness.

38-year-old Yogesh from Udaipur had COVID-19 with intense coughing. His chest had tightened, and it almost felt like he was going to have a heart attack. Using the techniques in this section gave him relief. It was also an eye-opener on how the mind can affect the body. Anxiety and fear worsen the symptoms, as most individuals do not understand what is happening to the body. Soft-tissue release of this section is the miracle that most individuals are looking for to rid themselves of this constant fear.

Soft-tissue release of this section takes precedence for those who also want improvements in their respiratory ailments.

Pectoralis Major and Minor

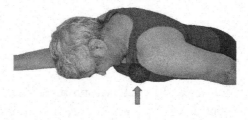

Pectoralis Major

Take a medium/hard ball and lie down on the floor on your stomach while targeting each painful, tight or tender area in the chest. Inhale deeply and, while you exhale, try to press deeper into the targeted area. Remember, the breath is what relaxes your tissue and allows the tool to penetrate deeper into the layers of soft tissue. This release is performed by pressing individual spots around the whole chest area. Staying with each spot till you cover the chest is an ideal way to get rid of symptoms. Be mindful of the ribs underneath the layers of tissue.

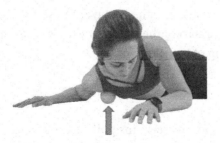

Pectoralis Minor

To dig into the pectoralis minor, place the ball close to the armpit and try rotating the torso on the same side while taking support of the opposite palm. The pec minor is a tighter, smaller, neglected muscle that is affected because of poor posture.

Subclavius

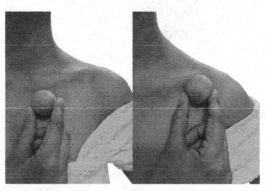

Start point   End point

Try and find hotspots right under your collarbone. While lying on the stomach, move in the direction along the collarbone in micro-movements. Breathe deeply into the hard/medium ball right from the start of the collarbone till you reach its end and the beginning of the shoulder.

Sternum

The breastbone may seem insignificant, but it can be the most painful area to touch. A hard squash ball or a soft crazy ball can be good options for this massage.

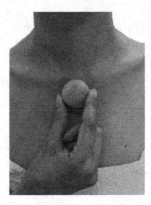

Top of the breast bone

Lie down on the stomach and keep the ball between the collarbones. Move the ball on top of the breast bone. Move downward to work directly on the breastbone.

After you reach the end of the breastbone, place the ball at the end between both ribs. Keep breathing deeply till the ball penetrates deep enough and you start feeling your breathing is effortless and wholesome. The ball must not be placed on top of the ribs but where you have soft tissue between the ribs.

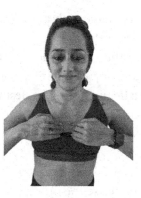

Then place the ball along the sides of the breast bone. Move along both the sides of the breastbone millimetre by millimetre really close to the bone till you reach the end. Breathe deeply into each spot.

Triceps, Biceps, Brachialis

Muscles that move the upper arm include the biceps and triceps. These areas must be checked, as triggers can set off pain in the shoulder, back, upper arm, forearm, and fingers.

Triceps

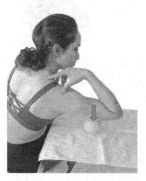

Sit on a chair next to a table with a hard ball right at the base of the elbow. To ensure the ball doesn't slip, you can use an anti-skid surface on the table under the ball. Lean into the elbow by using your body weight and push the ball into the triceps muscle. As a beginner, it is easiest to start this release work in the very centre of the muscle, moving upward a few inches before you reach the armpit. Release the trigger points one spot at a time.

Once you feel more confident, work slightly right and left of the muscle to release the outer and inner bands of the muscle. If the ball slips, use the other hand to support it.

Biceps

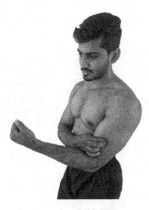

Use your fingers to pinch the bicep muscle. Feel the tight painful spots and apply constant pressure while palpating it a few times till you feel more at ease. Move along the whole area of the muscle from the top to the bottom, working each section bit by bit.

Brachialis

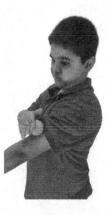

With this release you want to target the region under the shoulder till the elbow.

Support your arm on a table and rub a hard ball along the brachialis with the other hand. You can alternatively use your fingers to pinch the muscle like the biceps.

- **Stretches**

Rotator Cuff

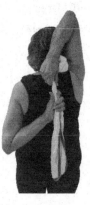

Use a towel or belt for this stretch. Place one arm behind and try pulling it higher with the other. You should feel a stretch in the shoulder. Hold the stretch for sixty seconds and repeat on the other side.

Latissimus Dorsi

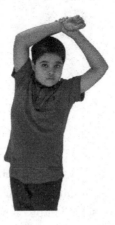

While seated, hold the wrist of one hand with the other. Lift the arm overhead and pull the wrist in the opposite direction. You should feel a stretch in the side of the body of the arm being pulled. Breathe deeply into the side, stretching while you hold it for sixty seconds. Repeat on the other side.

Chest

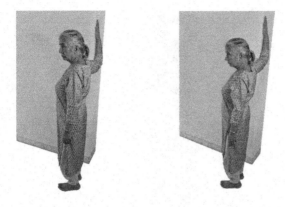

Image 1: Stand with your arm bent and forearm on the edge of a wall. Rotate your body in the other direction to feel the stretch in the chest on the side that has the arm on the wall. Hold it for twenty seconds.

Image 2: Repeat the same procedure as you slowly move slightly upward. Keep moving higher after every twenty seconds till the arm is high enough in a bent position. You can hold the stretch more at the angle that feels the tightest. Repeat this with the other arm to stretch the other side of the chest.

Triceps

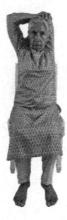

While seated, bring one arm up and grab the elbow with the other hand. Pull the elbow towards the centre of the head till you feel a stretch in the triceps. Hold it and breathe into it for sixty seconds and repeat it on the other arm.

Biceps

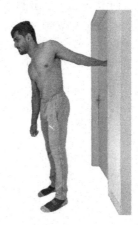

Grab a door handle with one arm and turn your body away so as to extend the arm completely, making sure the elbow doesn't bend. The arm should be positioned sideways, extending behind the body. Hold the stretch for 30–60 seconds. Repeat on the other hand.

Abdominals

- **Pain symptoms experienced**
  Burping, bladder pain, nausea and vomiting are some symptoms. Triggers in the abdomen are responsible for referred pain around the abdomen, groin, thigh and lower back.

- **Why and how this soft-tissue release can help you**
  Individuals with posterior pelvic tilt and anterior pelvic tilt can benefit from massaging the abdominals, especially if they suffer from lower-back pain.

  If you urinate frequently or experience urine retention, then check to see if release of myofascial triggers in the abdomen improve the symptoms. 28-year-old Veenu was regularly signing up for 'ab challenges' to get her ideal washboard flat abs. One day she started experiencing urinary tract infection (UTI) pains. Her abdomen was in a constant state of contraction because she was overdoing abdominal exercises. When she started performing soft-tissue releases in this section, she realized how tight and painful it really was. Besides the UTI, which settled immediately without any medication, she realized that the flat abs were really not worth the distress.

When you perform soft tissue release on the abdomen, you can improve your loss of appetite and gut-related issues, and also reduce your acid reflux. The gut is also responsible for cardiac symptoms, heartburn and cardiac arrhythmia, so relief from these issues is experienced right after the massage.

If you have respiratory issues, like an inability to take full breaths that causes anxiety because of diaphragm tightness, releasing the abdomen can help.

The feeling of a 'stitch in the side' while running or doing exercise can be eased out by the techniques described in this section.

• **Affected areas**

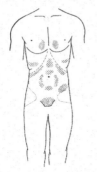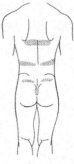

Check to see if you experience pain or any symptoms in these areas. It is always wise to club the release of this section with chest massage if your symptoms in the two sections overlap. After doing the release exercises, you may find your centre of gravity shifts, and walking may initially feel very different. *Your body may feel less anchored with a slight loss of stability,*

but it is crucial at this point to continue to maintain an ideal posture, engaging the core during all activities so as to not overcompensate elsewhere.

- **Tools**
  A medium/soft ball and a hardback book.

- **Soft-tissue release techniques**

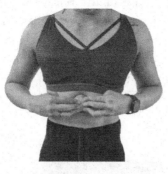

Start by placing a medium or soft ball right between the bones of the bottom ribs above the navel. If you are unsure, then take some practical guidance with Move Better Wellness to ensure you are using these techniques safely and with maximum benefit.

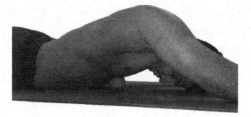

Lie down on the stomach with a soft or medium hard ball. Breathe deeply so you can go deeper without feeling discomfort. In case you do not feel any release, then place a hardback book between the ball and the floor. This intensifies the release, as the ball penetrates deeper.

Slowly inch down towards the navel and breathe into the next spot. Gradually move down until you reach the pubic bone.

The next phase of the release is to move 2 inches parallel to the centre under the last rib on the right. Gradually move down along this line, breathing and releasing inch by inch till you reach the hip bone.

Repeat this on the left.

This covers the entire area abdomen from the front.

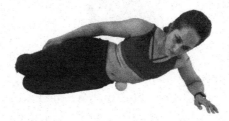

We now try to target the obliques from the side. Place the ball 2 inches away on the right side of the navel and turn slightly to the side, pushing the ball sideways into the abdomen. Explore tight spots in this region.

Repeat this on the left.

- **Stretches**

Mobility Cobras

This is a great stretch for the abdomen as well as for lower-back pain. It improves mobility in all segments of the spine.

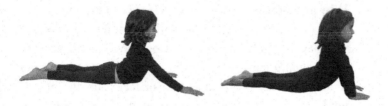

Lie down on the stomach with the palms placed on both sides of the head. Inhale, and on the exhale, lift the trunk into a cobra with straight arms. After a few seconds, lower the trunk back to the floor and place the palms an inch behind towards the shoulder. Repeat the stretch and keep inching down till your palms comfortably reach the chest. Feel a stretch in the abdomen.

Lower back, Buttocks, Hip and Hamstring

- **Pain symptoms experienced**
  Even though lower-back pain is globally the most common ailment today, before we rush into self-diagnosing our pains by labelling them as 'back pain' or 'sciatica', we must consider trigger points and tightness in the lower back, hip and buttock muscles, which may be contributing to our uneasiness. The lower-back muscles can be responsible for pain in the glutes and vice versa.

Besides our lifestyle and postural habits, foot and calf tightness and triggers can aggravate pain in the lower back.

Aches and pains in the lower-back, tailbone and buttock areas are symptoms.

- **Why and how this soft-tissue release can help you**

Your lower-back tightness will definitely ease out if you have an anterior or posterior pelvic tilt. If you are experiencing pain while sitting, lying down, getting out of a car, getting up from a chair or feel your hip locking while getting up after sitting, refer to these techniques. Sciatica pain and pain experienced while walking, lying down and getting out of bed can be released when this section is massaged alongside the hip, Iliotibial (IT) band, thigh, groin, calf, ankle and foot.

If you experience stiffness or discomfort or are stuck in a limited range in your dead-lifts and squats, then using this section is crucial.

Too much sitting causes stress on the musculature of the trunk. Thus, if you are regular with soft-tissue release, you will be able to maintain spinal health and mobility by avoiding early degeneration.

Children and adults who engage in high-impact sports are exposed to more load, which can stress out the lower back more than that of an average individual. This makes them more vulnerable to lower-back degeneration. Maintaining the strength and length in these regions is absolutely vital for sports-loving individuals.

Improvements in our daily posture, spinal stability, skill in our movements, combined with the maintenance techniques in this section, greatly reduce the chances of disc herniation, slipped discs, disc bulges and neural impingements that are as common as flu, even in 20-year-olds.

- **Affected areas**

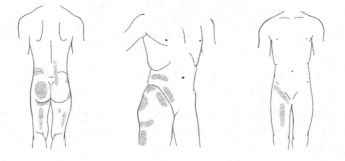

Check to see if you experience pain or any symptoms in these areas. Note that, besides soft-tissue release, these issues are best resolved with an adequate strengthening programme. Lower-back pains are complex to deal with and require professional help and guidance. For the best results, seek help from Move Better Wellness to guide you to troubleshoot your issues scientifically and safely, step by step.

- **Tools**
  - A peanut ball
  - A hard, round myofascial ball the size of a tennis ball

- **Soft-tissue release techniques**

Moving Along the Spine

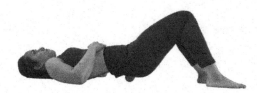

Use a peanut ball for this release while lying on your back. Start by placing the ball close to your tailbone and, with bent knees, roll the ball in micro-movements up and down. Ensure the gap in the peanut ball is always where your spinal bone fits and the two ends of the ball are alongside the spine and never directly on the spine. Travel upwards in micro-movements towards your lower back, with your buttocks touching the floor as you reach the lower back. Trigger points can occur anywhere along the spine.

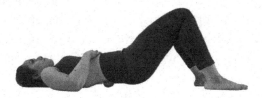

Travel further up till you reach the thoracic-lumbar junction which is located at the end of your ribcage. Mobilize this region by staying at one point and try to move the buttocks up and down. It can be quite painful, but it will release the most stubborn area in the spine.

You can move upwards towards the neck, covering all the regions of the mid-back and upper back. The best part of this release is that it automatically increases spinal flexibility.

After you are done, hug the knees into your chest for a minute.

Then turn the knees side to side to stretch the lower back.

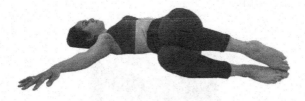

The paraspinal muscles are at a parallel distance away from the spine and the area just worked. Use a small, hard/medium ball to move two inches away from the spine. Start from either the right or left lower back, right above the glutes, and travel up to the bottom of the shoulder blades. You can work more parallel lines close to each other by rolling up and down and left and right on the tight spots.

Buttock and Hips

Gluteus maximus

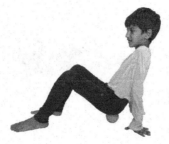

Use a hard, medium-sized ball and sit on it on one buttock. Roll the buttock in upward and downward movements. The idea is to target the entire length of the buttock. To reach other areas, such as the top portion of the buttock, you can lie down to push the ball in deeper.

Gluteus medius

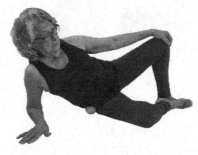

Lie down on your side and roll the ball under the side of the buttock. Stay at spots that feel tender, tight or painful and then flush out the muscle with larger rolling strokes.

Ilipsoas

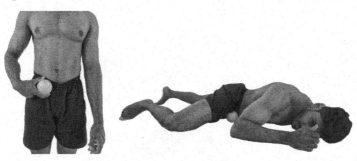

Take a medium-hard ball and place it above right on the inside of the hip bone. Lie down on the stomach and start by bending the knee. As you exhale, push the ball deep into the hip flexor and slowly extend the leg. Release the ball and bend the knee again to repeat this process multiple times, till you find a sense of ease setting in. Breathe to relax the muscles of the hip. If you have trouble bending the knee and lifting the leg up in a standing position, then this is what you need to focus on. Repeat this on the other leg.

Hamstrings

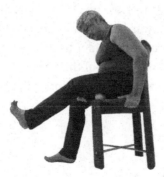

Take a small, hard ball and place it where the buttock bone ends. Use a chair with a hard surface or a wooden bench. Lean forward so that the ball digs into the top end of the hamstring. Extend your leg up and down till you feel that spot ease out. Then keep travelling inch by inch, covering the entire length of the leg, until you reach the topmost portion of the back of the knee. This releases the centre of the hamstring.

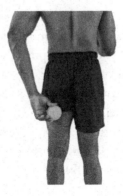

We want to target the *biceps femoris*, which is parallel to the centre that you just worked on. Move an inch and a half away from the centre towards the outer edge of the leg and start from the topmost portion under the glutes until you reach the topmost portion of the back of the knee.

The parallel line towards the inner thigh can be targeted in the same way.

- **Stretches**

Lower-Back Stretches

Our back muscles are connected with the abdominals and their integrity is balanced with right posture. If the abdominals are tight and over-exercised, it will tilt the lower-back muscles posteriorly, flattening out its natural curvature. If the lower-back muscles are over-exercised and tight due to our loading patterns and posture, it will increase the natural curvature of the lower back. Thus, it is crucial to maintain spinal integrity by using our back muscles effectively to lengthen the spine versus shortening it by compressing the musculature. The safe and effective ways to stretch the lower back are mentioned below, but it must be noted that *if we maintain good postural alignment, these stretches become redundant in daily life.* It is good to perform them after the release to restore the balance of the tissue and restore our posture.

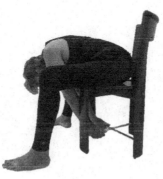

Sit on a chair with the legs apart. With an exhalation, slowly lower and sink into the chair, allowing the muscles of the entire back to relax. Breathe deeply.

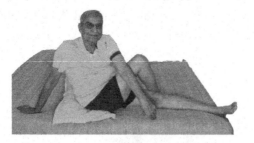

This stretch works well for the back as well as the glutes. Sit comfortably on the floor or a hard bed with one knee bent. Rotate the body to the side and place your elbow or arm over the bent knee. With every breath, try to increase the rotation if you are comfortable. Overdoing it will make it tight.

The standing rotations as well as chair rotations (refer to page 134 and 135) can also be performed.

Glutes

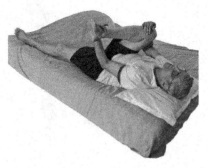

Lie down on the floor and hug one knee to the chest. Place one hand on top of the knee to pin it closer to the chest and the other hand on the ankle to draw it closer to the opposite side of the body. Breathe into this stretch as you hold it for a minute. In addition, you can point and flex the foot to flush out the nerves.

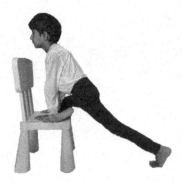

The standing pigeon stretch can be performed on a table at waist height or lower, depending on your ability to raise the leg comfortably. Senior citizens can use the edge of a bed, which is safer.

Place the leg at a height and try to maintain a 90-degree angle between the hip, knee and ankle. Slowly, lower the body towards the side of the knee as you breathe out and come up. Take another breath and lower the body in the centre and come up. Then on the side of the ankle. Repeat the stretch in all these three angles till you experience a sense of ease in the hip and glutes.

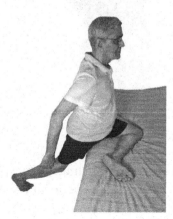

This is an alternative to the pigeon stretch. It can be performed by seniors or those with knee and hip limitations. Sit on a chair with one leg bent and the ankle on the thigh in the figure of four (4). Then rotate the body towards the knee, keeping the back straight. Lean forward till you feel a stretch in the hip/buttock. Keep the back very straight as you lean into the stretch. Then come up and lean forward in the centre. Stay till it eases out. Repeat this on the side of the ankle. Then perform all these three variations on the other leg.

Hamstrings

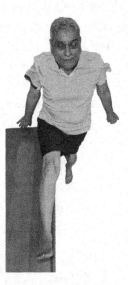

The lying down doorway stretch is the most relaxing stretch for the hamstring and is safe to perform even with back pain. Find a doorway where you can comfortably elevate one leg while resting the other on the floor. You can stay up for 10 minutes on each leg if it is comfortable. After a few minutes, see if the muscle has lengthened and move the leg higher to increase the intensity of the stretch. You should be able to sustain it for a longer period of time, so start out comfortably. Try to relax, breathe and disconnect the mind.

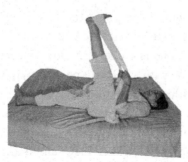

If you are unable to sit on the floor, then use a belt or stole to elevate the leg for a minute on both legs.

Knee, Thigh, IT Band and Groin/Inner Thigh

- **Pain symptoms experienced**

  If you experience pain in the knees and legs without lower-back pain, then you can troubleshoot directly with this section.

  Often, overall pain in the lower limbs is accompanied with pain in the hip and groin. The hip and groin are companions of the legs which are often overlooked and not maintained.

- **Why and how this soft-tissue release can help you**

  Professionals such as doctors, wedding planners, photographers, chefs and other individuals who have long hours of standing and staying on their feet find relief when releases in this section are combined with those of the calf, ankle and foot.

  If you are struggling with stiff legs, can't cross them while sitting or comfortably raise them, or if you have suddenly started limping, then you will find instant improvements using these techniques.

Improvements are seen in individuals with mild knee pain or those with strained knees or pain while climbing stairs. Buckling of knees and back of the knee pain reduce.

Many regular runners, walkers and individuals into cardiovascular fitness activities experience IT band syndrome, which is easily maintained and avoided with regular use of this section.

If your sport involves a lot of lower limb activity, such as cycling or playing football, then this section maintains the mobility as well as repairs, restores and rejuvenates the lower limbs.

Frequent travellers and desk-bound individuals will find comfort and improvement in their quality of life, if the releases in this section are used periodically.

- **Affected areas**

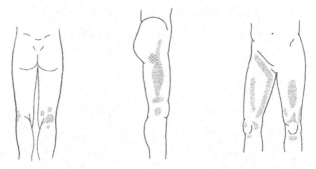

Check to see if you experience pain or any symptoms in these areas. Even after performing these techniques, if your pains persist beyond two weeks, consider some professional evaluation with Move Better Wellness.

- **Tools**
    - Hard balls of various sizes
    - Hardback book/yoga block
    - A rolling pin

- **Soft-tissue release techniques**

Thigh

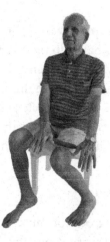

Take a rolling pin and target the middle of the thigh by digging the rolling pin deeply. Start at the top of the knee and travel all the way up, bit by bit, till you reach the upper thigh. Push into spots that feel tight, tender or painful. This frees up the rectus femoris muscle. Repeat this on the other leg.

Work the same way by targeting the outer edge of your thigh. This is the *vastus lateralis* muscle of the thigh. Repeat this on the other leg.

Iliotibial band/IT Band

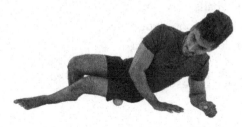

Lie down on your side, placing a medium/hard ball on the side of the thigh. Push the ball into tight or tender spots and wait there till the pain eases out. Then roll the ball to smoothen out the surface of the sides of the thigh. Pay attention to this band of tissue, as it is not a muscle and cannot be stretched effectively. The best way to maintain this area and avoid knee pain is using this soft-tissue release technique.

Inner Thigh and Groin

The adductors are a group of muscles that when tight, can alter our walking, sitting and moving. This region is tender and does not feel pleasant on release. Nevertheless, triggers must be reduced as they can wreak havoc in our movement.

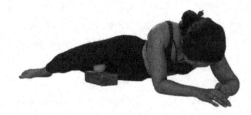

Take a yoga block/hardback book with a medium/hard ball. If this region is very sensitive for you, start with a softer ball and gradually progress to a harder one. Extend the leg out with the knee bent, and push into the inner thigh which is closest to the knee. this can be performed on the floor without a book or yoga block but the height raises the leg and makes this release easier. Try moving the ball in micro-movements up and down and left and right. Travel upward along the inner thigh till you reach the groin. Don't forget to breathe deeply.

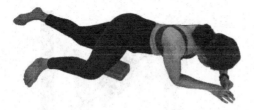

At first, this may seem time-consuming and you may be clumsy, but every time you practise, it will get easier.

Back of the Knee

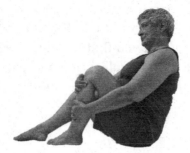

Take a hard squash ball for this. You are trying to create some space in the knee joint with this technique. Push the ball deep inside the back of the knee and bend it. Hug the knee in and hold it tight. The ball should be pushed directly into the skin, without any clothing obstructing it. You can do this anywhere, anytime to reduce knee pain instantly!

• **Stretches**

Thigh

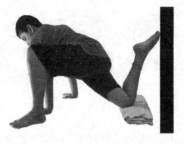

Go down on the floor and bend the knee as illustrated while placing it close to a wall. You can alternatively use the bed if you can't go down on the floor. Your shin should touch the wall or the edge of the bed. Place the other leg forward and both your hands on one side. Feel a stretch in the thigh. Try and hold this till you find the muscle easing out. If it doesn't, go back to the rolling pin and dig into the spots that feel tight and stretch it again. This may take a few days to feel good.

Inner Thigh

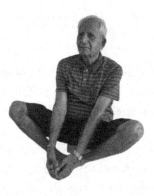

There are many spots you cannot stretch in the inner thigh. The butterfly is the most commonly used stretch that helps ease out parts of the groin and inner thigh muscle. However, targeting spots using the release technique is far superior.

Sit on a cushion/yoga block with bent knees. Place the soles of your feet close together so they touch. With a straight back, see if you can move forward. Keep breathing and hold the stretch till you feel a sense of ease. Keep leaning forward with a straight back to increase the intensity of the stretch. Areas of the hip and groin take time to ease out. Aggressive painful stretching only creates further tightness. I would recommend at least five minutes in this position to feel a sense of ease. If you are used to performing this stretch dynamically by lifting the knees, then do that to begin with.

Calf, Ankle and Feet

- **Pain symptom experienced**
  Swelling of the feet, difficulty in standing and walking, pain in the top of the foot and back of the foot, heel pain,

pain in the ankle and back of the knee, calf and shin pain, shin splints, plantar fasciitis and foot cramps are the areas you want to treat with this section.

- **Why and how this soft-tissue release can help you**
  If you have a lot of foot problems, fallen arches, bow legs, bunions, knock knees, hammer toes or any deformity of the foot, then this section is your lifeline.

  This section is a must for individuals of all ages to maintain and prevent any pain in the legs. If you want to keep walking pain-free as long as you live, then maintaining these areas is crucial.

  Those who have issues with their gait see improvements with regular use of this massage section along with a change in their posture.

  Those who wish to prepare to walk effortlessly on inclined surfaces, uphill, downhill and on uneven surfaces must consider performing these before they begin.

  Stiff toes and immobile ankles can be opened up with this section. Individuals with knee pain also experience relief when they troubleshoot with this section in addition to the soft-tissue techniques of the knee.

  If you stand a lot, then indulging in these releases every day pampers those feet that need their due attention to feel good the next day.

- **Affected areas**

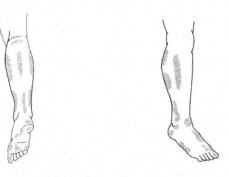

Check to see if you experience pain or any symptoms in these areas. Troubleshooting all these muscle groups together is essential to experience relief from any minor or major pain.

- **Tools**
  - Balls of various degrees of hardness
  - A wooden/aluminum stick
  - A rolling pin

- **Soft-tissue release techniques**

Calf

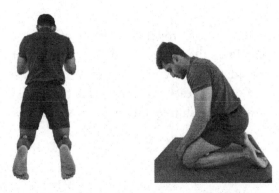

Take two golf balls or anything that is of the same size and hardness. You can sit on a bed or on the floor. Place the balls close to the back of both the knees and try to sit back on the heels.

If it is very painful, lower yourself only as much as you can. After this point eases out, place the balls slightly lower and again sit back on the heels to release the lower end of the calf muscle. Keep inching lower till you reach the end of the calves. It is essential that the calf release isn't ignored if you have pain in the sole of your foot. Triggers in the calf are responsible for foot cramps and pain.

Tibialis Anterior

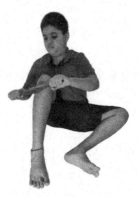

Take a rolling pin and roll it on the front of the leg close to the shin bone. Press the rolling pin slightly off the bone towards the outer side. Start under the knee in small movements up and down till you reach the ankle. This helps ankle mobility and recovery from shin-splints and stress fractures.

Ankle

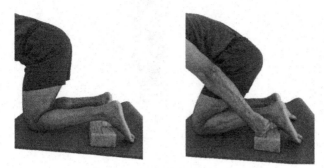

Image 1: Take a hard ball and place it on the top of the ankle. Push the ball into the ankle joint against a hard surface, keeping the foot off the edge.

Image 2: While holding the ball with your fingers, sit back into the heel to increase pressure on the ankle. Then move the foot up and down to open out the ankle joint. This creates space and frees up restrictions in the ankle.

Foot

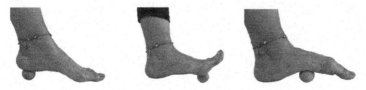

Take a medium-soft ball and step on it with the arch of the foot. Push it in and roll it all along the arch, heel and forefoot. This eases out the sole of the foot.

You can also rub a medium-soft or soft ball on the top of the foot if you experience pain there.

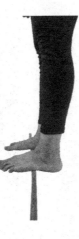

In addition to this, you can stand on a wooden or aluminium stick, pushing your heels first into it. You don't need to set aside time for this, as it can be done at your standing desk while working or while you cook or watch television. After you feel the pain in your heels has reduced, slowly move lower, inching towards the forefoot. Stay longer at points that cause the most pain. To feel like you have a fresh pair of feet, perform this routine daily. It also makes standing long hours more comfortable and reduces swelling.

- **Stretches**

Calf

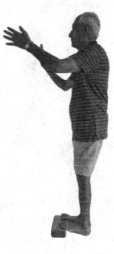

Place a yoga block 4 inches away from a wall. Then place your toes as high as possible on the block with the heels touching the floor. Then lean the body into the wall, without jutting out the hip. Make sure the heels don't lift off the floor. Hold till the stretch in the calves has eased out.

Ankle

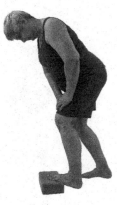

Place one foot on the yoga block. Then support your hands on the knee and push the knee forward without lifting the ankle off the floor. You should feel a stretch at the back of the ankle and at the Achilles' tendon.

Tibialis Anterior

This is a simple position you can get into effortlessly anywhere and anytime. It eases out the shin and increases ankle mobility. Simply sit with one leg extended behind with the top of the foot facing the ground. Gently press the foot into the ground till you feel a stretch. Then release after a few seconds and repeat multiple rounds of this, keeping the foot at the same angle.

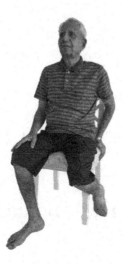

You can change the angle of the foot by turning it inwards and outwards to get into different areas of the top part of the foot and ankle.

Arch of the Foot

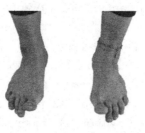

Stretching and maintaining suppleness in the arch of the foot is very simple for those with fallen arches. Lift the big toe up as many times as you can while gripping the other toes into the floor. Perform this multiple times during the day to ease out pain in the arch of the foot.

7

Wellness for Desk-Bound Individuals

A comprehensive approach to employee quality of life needs to be adopted so that they can deliver top-notch performance while thinking of their long-term well-being. Most approaches ignore the following factors:

- Most individuals are sedentary twenty-three hours a day and move just an hour. This makes them struggle with the basics of human function and health.
- A desk-bound individual has limited range of motion in the joints and stiff muscles that are the consequence of inadequate hydration and poor posture. Efforts to increase mobility without addressing the causes are of little use.
- Stored muscle tension and emotions that are not removed from the physical body cause breathing limitations, which lead to anxiety and nervous tension. The state of the body detracts from the value of the courses undertaken

to improve mental health. Troubleshooting the physical body thus becomes a pre-requisite for mental health.

- Basic movement mechanics of spinal stability, sitting, bending, standing, walking are untrained, thus neutralizing any benefit derived from fitness activities.

General fitness and corporate programmes don't provide solutions to these causes and their effects. Employee welfare can be addressed only by including all these above aspects into a programme that focuses on the basics of health and well-being.

These techniques must be used by desk-bound individuals to add mobility solutions to their daily life. Besides combating pain, the solutions provided make the brain alert and promote relaxation in the body. None of these divert the already preoccupied mind while working and can be used every day to increase blood circulation. These self-care techniques counter the effects of daily life stress and come with many benefits.

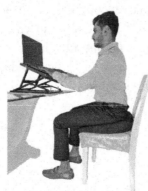

- Sitting with a wedge cushion keeps the spine erect and brain alert. The spine can stay erect longer without a back support and feel no fatigue. This is half the battle won as mobility isn't compromised.

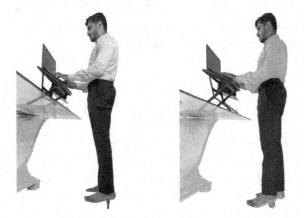

- Using a stick/rolling pin or ball under the foot at a standing desk prevents the fatigue (from standing), enhances posture and increases blood circulation. This is a position that encourages brain activity, improves concentration and creativity, and charges up the brain with ideas, increasing output. This is also a great way to increase NEAT* calories for those individuals who have excessive sedentary hours.

---

* NEAT (Non-exercise activity thermogenesis) refers to the calories we burn during the day apart from our exercise hours. An example of burning NEAT calories can be standing, waiting in queues, walking in the house, cooking, washing dishes, cleaning, shopping, driving, indulging in hobbies that are not sedentary, etc.

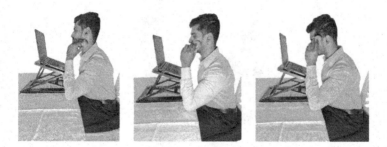

- Rubbing a myofascial ball along the sides of the neck, jaw and head is an anxiety and stress-buster that increases circulation in the head and eyes. The entire action is inconspicuous!

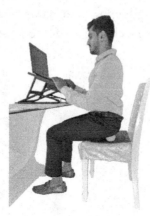

- Myofascial release for the glutes keeps the hip mobile. Simply place a hard to medium ball under the buttocks. To prevent the ball from sinking into your chair you can use a hard placemat under the ball. This technique also massages the glutes and increases blood circulation in the area.

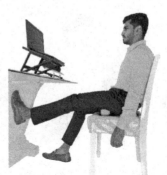

- Myofascial release for hamstrings ensures you will never have to experience back pain because of sitting! Imagine the magic of lengthening your hamstrings while you sit. For details on the technique, refer to page 205.

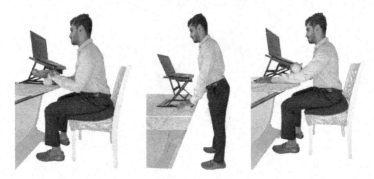

- Wrist, palm and forearm release with a ball not only improves mobility in the wrist, fingers and forearm, but it counters the stress on the palms, fingers, wrist and forearms caused by using devices.

  Image 1: Place a ball under the wrist with your palms facing upwards. Place the other hand on top to put a gentle pressure and mobilize the wrist by moving it up and down. This instantly gives relief from wrist pain.

Image 2: While standing, lean forward and put your body weight on a medium to hard ball placed under your palms. The pressure will automatically make your palm and fingers feel light. Those with carpal tunnel will get some ease from this simple release technique.

Image 3: Place a hard to medium ball on one forearm and dig into various areas of the forearm. This gives instantly relief for those suffering from tennis elbow.

8

Movement and Mental Health

Movement should be approached like life—with enthusiasm, joy and gratitude—for movement is life and life is movement and we get out of it what we put into it.—Ron Fletcher

While everyone seems to understand that exercise has multiple benefits and talks about it ad nauseam, most people don't really know the why and how.

Many of the psychological benefits[1] that are experienced with movement come from the 'exercise high'. A high can be expressed as euphoria or joy, which is a love of something without the side effects of addiction. People comment that their worries, stress and anxiety all fade away in that euphoria.

These psychological changes occur thanks to the endocannabinoid system (ECS). The ECS is a biochemical substance similar to the cannabis drug, so when we get a 'high', it is not an endorphin rush but the ECS that is responsible for the relaxed post-exercise feeling. Endocannabinoids are naturally produced by the body and increase during exercise.

A lot of research is done today to find out the benefits ECS has on general well-being and how it reduces or controls pain. The ECS comprises a powerful biological organization of multiple controls that affect mood, inflammation and pain and thus, has an analgesic effect on the body, along with other benefits to neurological aspects of the central and peripheral nervous system.[2] This is why many runners experience their pain vanishing with persistent running—the ECS system acts as a natural painkiller.

One outcome of regular exercise is generalized well-being, but the ECS is responsible for exerting control on multiple systems throughout our life. This includes anti-ageing,[3] which is why dermatologists prescribe exercise.

The ECS system controls appetite and positively influences the systemic energy metabolism. These dietary factors alter the responses of the brain,[4] which is why nutritionists prescribe exercise.

The reproductive system is also influenced by the ECS,[5] where it affects folliculogenesis, oocyte maturation and ovarian endocrine secretion. In addition, the ECS affects oviductal embryo transport and implantation. This is why gynaecologists prescribe exercise for women and girls with pregnancy or menstrual issues.

There is a complex interplay between the ECS and the hypothalamic-pituitary-ovarian axis (HPA), as well as between the ECS and steroid hormone production and secretion. The immune system is affected by the HPA. This explains why exercise works as a stress buster that strengthens immunity and prevents illness.[6]

When we move everyday with persistence, it neutralizes and cancels the brain's response to everyday mental and emotional stress. Stress is an everyday battle so we need the movement pill every day to negate its effects. This is why the general physician prescribes exercise too. *Immunity against disease isn't a thrice-a-week ritual. The stress battle can be fought every day in some way, either by improving mobility or by improving posture or by adding strength or self-myofascial release or simply challenging the brain and body with periodic movement breaks.*

The ECS is also known for its positive impact on multiple sclerosis, Alzheimer's disease and amyotrophic lateral sclerosis.[7] It has an influence on memory function.[8] You now know why neurologists prescribe the movement pill. Regular cardiovascular exercise can spark the growth of new blood vessels and new brain cells that keep nourishing the brain, improving brain performance and preventing cognitive decline.[9]

Exercise improves cognition, which has important implications for improving academic performance in children and college students, improving adult productivity, preserving cognitive function in old age, preventing or treating certain neurological disorders and improving overall quality of life. Children who move have increased learning and memory function compared to those who just study. The movement pill is often prescribed to a distracted mind that has difficulty sticking to one task and completing it. Movement can be the easiest way to encourage the mentally challenged and children suffering from ADHD. They are known to cope better and gain from neurological changes that result from movement.

Persistence with Movement

Now that we understand the multiple benefits of the ECS system, what is the best way during exercise to release endocannabinoids? What can we do to aid this process? Running and dancing are not the only ways to release endocannabinoids. Many movements can lead to a 'high'. An interesting finding by researcher David A. Raichlen was that the release of endocannabinoids during exercise is modulated by intensity.[10] If you run or move too fast, they don't get released into the bloodstream. Neither does the release occur if you are too slow. *But a moderately challenging physical activity, sustained over a period of 20–30 minutes, is enough. Moderately challenging movement, sustained daily with 'persistence', is the key factor that is responsible for all the positive outcomes we are awarded with, be it physical or psychological.*

Another study found a correlation between the runner's high and state of flow.[11] The way to induce this state is to find a balance between the challenge and skill of any activity. An activity that is too challenging or not sufficiently challenging makes the individual disinterested and doesn't induce the mental state of flow. Concentration requires a moderate challenge that holds the attention of the individual, thus inducing states of satisfaction and joy. This sense of satisfaction will always propel an individual to pursue their movement goals with more persistence.

Regular movement increases and adds to our optimism—provided it is 'sustained persistently'. It neutralizes and cancels the brain's stress response if pursued on a daily basis. This doesn't mean we add another stress element of having to move every day in our life—we have enough stress as it is. Stressing over something that is meant to give us joy and freedom from stress isn't the right approach. The mindset should be to increase our ability to stick to our tasks, goals and passions slowly but surely, with consistency.

Various studies have shown that perseverance is an essential quality for success in life.[12] It often precedes aptitude and raw talent and is an accurate predictor of success. It strengthens our ability to learn from failure and increases willpower when we try and try again and never accept defeat.[13] If you want to develop a strong will and increase perseverance, adding movement to your life will help. *Persevering is easy for an individual who falls in love with and marries movement.* We can learn from the miracle inside us—our heartbeat. The heart beats 60–70 times per minute, awake or asleep, day or night—it persists. When our heart beats, it's working hard, it's moving constantly. With its persistent activity, everything in the body comes alive.

Research proves that frequent exercisers have higher levels of self-efficacy and persistence and consequently experience greater facilitation towards attaining both exercise and non-exercise goals.[14] *If we persist in movement, we persist in life towards all endeavours and that becomes our personality.* Being inconsistent and not feeling good enough are not traits of an athlete or an achiever. *Persistent effort never goes to waste, even if the results don't show up instantly. Self-growth is the best outcome we achieve as a result of our persistent labouring.*

It is not about the success of winning a gold medal in a short race. The wise long-term investments of mental evolution, which come with sound choices, create wealth.

Movement gains are long-term mental and psychological gains, not short-term gains.

Success and failure both give life meaning and purpose as each comes with its own lessons. This is how people with depression, asthma and broken bodies have risen to health and freedom, and this is how great inventions happen. *Pleasure and satisfaction don't come just from outcomes, but from the experiences prior to the outcome. It is these prior experiences that add meaning and value to life, not success or failure.*

Intensifying Deep Focus with Movement

Everyone talks about the benefits of meditation and breathing to combat stress and anxiety and to increase concentration, but there is an equal amount of research that proves movement does the same. We have seen how persistence of movement at a moderate intensity releases and activates the ECS, which induces deep focus, which in turn is responsible for psychological changes in a person. Many athletes experience a state of flow, in which they are completely absorbed in an activity that is intrinsically self-rewarding. It is the merging of action and awareness, centring of attention, loss of self-consciousness, feeling of control and distortion of time. Of course, a clear goal is the prerequisite for inducing flow.[15]

A clear goal, combined with persistence, makes the mover's experience of movement itself a meditation. Attention during meditation is directed inwards, but the states of flow experienced during movement are directed outward to the task at hand. Many find meditating a challenge, as moving attention inward can be tough—this is where movement can help.

The joy-induced states from being in flow with movement acts more like a preventive element to bad moods. *People meditate because they are anxious and depressed. But why wait to get into those moods in the first place when you can move to feel better instantly?* When we develop a deep connection with movement, we don't use movement to overcome bad moods or any other purpose—we move because it provides uninhibited joy. *Just as our thoughts exist persistently during waking hours, so should movement. When our thoughts and movements work alongside each other, they balance each other out.*

The prime mental states of being joyful, positive and active are an outcome of daily effort. If one is persistently focused, one doesn't need meditation. *Persistence is activity and deep focus. Thus, one does not need meditation, since persistence itself is the meditation!*

Optimism, satisfaction, joy, self-efficacy, persistence, being a go-getter, having the right attitude towards success and failure, increased attention and concentration, as well as balancing the effects of stress are all the mental benefits of movement and add significant value and purpose to life.

Epilogue

Am I Adapting to Pain or
Adapting to Better Function?

We humans are constantly adapting. As homo sapiens, we adapted from standing on four legs to standing on two, from sitting and sleeping on floors to sitting on chairs and sleeping on mattresses. The current human is walking daily to increase the quality of health, but if it leaves one with pain instead, is the movement really adding to the quality of one's health? By pushing our body through pain signals to keep moving (or do nothing), are we adapting the body to pain or are we pushing the body to adapt to better function? Are we adapting to fallen arches and to the use of arch supports, or are we adapting to restoring the natural arch of the foot? Am I adapting to reduced lung function with the inefficient postures and the poor use of technology? Am I adapting the body to advance in health, just as technology has advanced? Am I adapting my cells to decreased hydration? Am I adapting my bones to unequal load? With the use of painkillers and medicines, are we adapting to simply managing symptoms or are we adapting to continued dysfunction? Are we adapting our spines to disc degeneration and herniation by accepting and adapting to the bucket seats in airplanes, cars and modern furniture?

When I am trying to mimic a fitness influencer or achieve a body shape, I need to ask myself these questions—am I doing it to improve health and function? Am I doing it to get better at movement? Is what I am doing now sustainable? What body shapes am I adapting to? Without these aims, we can do the fancy routines prescribed by new-age fitness gurus or simply stick to the mundane fitness choices that are in our comfort zone, and keep oscillating between pain, inadequate function and new-year resolutions and goals that are never achieved.

Am I counterbalancing life with wisdom and determination in my pursuit for optimal health and efficiency?

Sustaining our current movements and continuously getting better at them requires us to first decondition poor movement habits. This is a lifelong programme in self-maintenance and awareness that will push us to better levels of sustained movement health and function.

Everyone who moves is an athlete. This includes a nurse or physiotherapist who pick up patients, a parent who carries and plays with their child, climbing the stairs of your duplex, carrying our own luggage while travelling or your heavy shopping bags from the supermarket or picking up heavy utensils in the kitchen. *Everyone is an athlete during some part of the day. The question is—are you a natural athlete?*

Natural athletes function with ease, quickly adapt to their environmental load and never withdraw from movement or complain about it. The term 'weekend warrior' needs to be replaced with the concept of 'natural warrior'.

Adding more movement to life after better quality of movement is easy. But if I perceive movement as a necessity, it stops becoming fun. Getting in and out of positions and using the body in different positions with the best possible mechanics should be associated with *fun* and *activity*. We should not move because we think 'it is good for me and has to be done'. It is a chance we can use to connect with ourselves through the body and understand where we lack courage, hope and determination. This is because the way we perceive movement is invariably the same outlook we have towards life. Rarely have we seen competitive athletes with a grim outlook towards life! To move better is to move like a natural athlete!

I hope this book has helped remove many misconceptions and fears regarding your health and well-being. The book doesn't end here. It's only the beginning of new heights to be scaled in movement and fitness. As a human race, we have been progressing through the millenniums, each era bringing about changes in lifestyle and sociophysical factors. Time and again, the challenges have been met in the most ingenious ways—that's what development is all about. We grow from less to more, from sufficient to efficient and finally to optimum. But the optimum is not a static point—it is an ever-ascending goal. If we continuously move better with the well-researched techniques documented in this book, we have most certainly arrived at a new height from where we can take off to even higher levels.

Welcome aboard! Please share this book and recommend it to others who would like to stay pain-free and move better. The speedy results of these techniques have improved the long-term health of so many individuals. If you're a parent, be a role model for your child and other family members and friends by adopting superior movement habits.

Acknowledgements

My name may be placed on the cover as the author of this book, but in truth I am only a tiny element that helped create it. The co-creators of this book are—

The Universe and my Guru.

I am grateful to my wonderful clients, who have given me a chance to serve them and learn life's invaluable lessons. A treasure trove of information comes from their experiences in illness and overcoming it. This wisdom will continue to stay alive for generations, in the lives, minds and hearts of all those who will learn about it in this book and use it.

I am lucky to have had the support of my wonderful parents who helped with this book, and a sister who has been inspirational in teaching me to stand when I could sit, walk when I could stand and run when I could walk.

I am indebted to Shoba Kirpalaney for all her valuable insights.

I thank Gray Cook, Esther Gokhale, Katy Bowman and Kelly Starrett for being a source of inspiration and making the world a better place with their contributions.

This book has only been possible because of the support of my literary agent Kanishka Gupta, Tarini Uppal and everyone at Penguin who believed in it, voted for it and have actively worked to publish and spread this awareness. Last but not the least, I thank the suffering I went through, as it gave me an education in lifelong well-being and introduced me to numerous teachers whose timely lessons taught me what I know today.

Notes

Preface

1. World Health Organization (WHO), 'Musculoskeletal Health', 14 July 2022, https://www.who.int/news-room/fact-sheets/detail/musculoskeletal-conditions.
2. Eileen M. Crimmins, 'Lifespan and Health Span: Past, Present, and Promise', *Gerontologist*, NCBI (2015), https://www.ncbi.nlm.nih.gov/pmc/articles/PMC4861644/, last accessed on 6 February 2023.

Chapter 1: Moving Better before Moving More

1. 'Sedentary Life's, the other global epidemic', World Bank, 15 October 2014, https://www.worldbank.org/en/news/feature/2014/10/15/vidas-sedentarias-la-otra-epidemia-global, last accessed on 6 February 2023.
2. Goodreads.com, 'Lou Holtz quotes', https://www.goodreads.com/quotes/21657-it-s-not-the-load-that-breaks-you-down-it-s-the, last accessed 6 April 2023.

Chapter 2: Posture

1. Claudia Hammond, 'Is crossing your legs bad for you?', BBC Future, 14 October 2015, https://www.bbc.com/future/article/20151013-is-crossing-your-legs-bad-for-you, last accessed on 6 February 2023.

2. Byung Joon Lee, et al., 'The effects of sitting with the right leg crossed on the trunk length and pelvic torsion of healthy individuals', *Journal of Physical Therapy Science*, November 2016, 28(11): 3162–64, https://www.ncbi.nlm.nih.gov/pmc/articles/PMC5140821/, last accessed on 6 February 2023.

3. Md Abu Bakar Siddiq, 'Wallet Neuritis – An Example of Peripheral Sensitization', *Current Rheumatology Reviews*, December 2018, 14(3): 279–83, https://www.ncbi.nlm.nih.gov/pmc/articles/PMC6204659/, last accessed on 6 February 2023.

4. '3 surprising risks of poor posture', *Harvard Health Publishing*, 15 February 2021, https://www.health.harvard.edu/staying-healthy/3-surprising-risks-of-poor-posture, last accessed on 6 February 2023.

5. Michelle Brandt, 'The health risks of high heels', *Scope: Stanford Medicine*, 25 January 2012, https://scopeblog.stanford.edu/2012/01/25/the-health-risks-of-high-heels/, last accessed on 6 February 2023.

6. Mohammad Zabetipour, et al., 'The Impacts of Open/closed Body Positions and Postures on Learners' Moods', *Mediterranean Journal of Social Sciences*, 6(2), S1 2015, https://www.mcser.org/journal/index.php/mjss/article/view/6002, last accessed on 6 February 2023.

7. '4.1 Principles and functions of non-verbal communication', in *Communication in the Real World*, University of Minnesota, M Libraries, https://open.lib.umn.edu/communication/chapter/4-1-principles-and-functions-of-nonverbal-communication/, last accessed on 6 February 2023.

8.   Amy Cuddy, 'Your body language may shape who you are', Ted Talk, https://www.ted.com/talks/amy_cuddy_your_body_language_may_shape_who_you_are?language=en, last accessed on 6 February 2023; Lynne Franklin, 'Reading minds through body language' Tedx Talk, https://www.youtube.com/watch?v=W3P3rT0j2gQ, last accessed on 6 February 2023.

9.   Lisa Owens Viani, 'Good posture is important for physical and mental health', San Francisco State University State News, 15 December 2017, https://news.sfsu.edu/news-story/good-posture-important-physical-and-mental-health, last accessed on 6 February 2023.

10. Erik Peper, et al., 'How Posture Affects Memory Recall and Mood, Project: The effect of posture on health', *Biofeedback*, 45(2): 36–41, April 2017, https://www.researchgate.net/publication/321348063_How_Posture_Affects_Memory_Recall_and_Mood, last accessed on 6 February 2023.

11. Erik Peper, 'Posture affects memory recall and mood', Pepper Perspective, 25 November 2017, https://peperperspective.com/2017/11/25/posture-affects-memory-recall-and-mood/.

12. Erik Peper, et al., 'How Posture Affects Memory Recall and Mood, Project: The Effect of Posture on Health', *Biofeedback*.

13. WonYang Kang, 'Comparison of anxiety and depression status between office and manufacturing job employees in a large manufacturing company: a cross sectional study', *Annals of Occupational and Environmental Medicine*, 28:47, 15 September 2016, last accessed on 6 February 2023.

14. The Alexander Lowen Foundation, 'What is Bioenergetics Analysis?', https://www.lowenfoundation.org/what-is-bioenergetics, last accessed on 6 April 2023.

15. Justin Leong and Shahid Akhter, 'There may be over 50 million people with sleep apnoea in India', *ET Health World*, 17 May 2019, https://health.economictimes.indiatimes.com/news/industry/there-may-be-over-50-million-people-with-sleep-

apnea-in-india-justin-leong/69366735, last accessed on 6 February 2023.

16. Ju-Yeon Jung, et al., 'Investigation on the Effect of Oral Breathing on Cognitive Activity Using Functional Brain Imaging', *PubMed*, 29 May 2021, https://pubmed.ncbi.nlm.nih. gov/34072444/, last accessed on 6 February 2023.

Chapter 3: Relearning Our Foundational Movement Principles

1. *Journal of Occupational Health*, 61(3): 227–234, May 2019, https://www.ncbi.nlm.nih.gov/pmc/articles/PMC6499348/.

2. *IOSR Journal of Dental and Medical Sciences* 3(2):8-12, January 2012, https://www.researchgate.net/publication/269753717_ Incidence_And_Study_of_Occupational_Factors_Associated_ With_Low_Back_Pain_In_Dentists_In_Pune_Region_ India.

3. '3 surprising risks of poor posture', *Harvard Health Publishing*, 15 February 2021, https://www.health.harvard.edu/staying- healthy/3-surprising-risks-of-poor-posture, last accessed on 6 February 2023.

4. Thomas Trojian, et al., 'Plantar Fasciitis', *AFP Journal* 99(12): 744–50, 15 June 2019, https://www.aafp.org/pubs/ afp/issues/2019/0615/p744.html, last accessed on 6 February 2023.

5. Yi-Lang Chen, et al., 'Posture and Time Arrangement Influence Shank Circumference Reduction When Performing Leg Raising Exercise', *International Journal of Environmental Research and Public Health*, 17(16): 5735, August 2020, https://www.ncbi. nlm.nih.gov/pmc/articles/PMC7460006/, last accessed on 6 February 2023.

6. Jessica Gross, 'Walking meetings? 5 surprising thinkers who swore by them', TED Blog, 29 April 2013, https://blog.ted.

com/walking-meetings-5-surprising-thinkers-who-swore-by-them/, last accessed on 6 February 2023.

7. 'Stanford study finds walking improves creativity', Stanford News, 24 April 2014, https://news.stanford.edu/2014/04/24/walking-vs-sitting-042414/, last accessed on 6 February 2023.

8. Marily Oppezzo and Daniel L. Schwartz, 'Give Your Ideas Some Legs: The Positive Effect of Walking on Creative Thinking', *Journal of Experimental Psychology Learning Memory and Cognition*, 40(4), April 2014, https://www.researchgate.net/publication/261768023_Give_Your_Ideas_Some_Legs_The_Positive_Effect_of_Walking_on_Creative_Thinking, last accessed on 6 February 2023.

9. Viraj N. Gandbhir, et al., 'Trendelenburg Gait', *NCBI*, May 2022, https://www.ncbi.nlm.nih.gov/books/NBK541094/#:~:text=A%20trendelenburg%20gait%20is%20an,the%20contralateral%20side%20while%20walking, last accessed on 6 February 2023.

10. Brent S. Russell, 'The effect of high-heeled shoes on lumbar lordosis: A narrative review and discussion of the disconnect between Internet content and peer-reviewed literature', *Journal of Chiropractic Medicine*, 9(4): 166–73, December 2010, https://www.ncbi.nlm.nih.gov/pmc/articles/PMC3206568/#:~:text=High%20heel%20shoes%20increase%20the%20forward%20curve%20of%20the%20low%20back.%E2%80%9D&text=%E2%80%9CWhenever%20you%20wear%20high%20heels,curve%20in%20your%20low%20back.%E2%80%9D&text=%E2%80%9CHigh%20heeled%20shoes%20can%20dramatically,lordosis)%20of%20the%20low%20back, last accessed on 6 February 2023.

11. Faith Heaton Jolley, 'Study shows the ways flip-flops damage feet', KSL News, 15 July 2013, https://www.ksl.com/article/26012248/study-shows-the-ways-flip-flops-damage-feet, last accessed on 6 February 2023.

12. Simon Franklin, et al., 'Barefoot vs common footwear: A systematic review of the kinematic, kinetic and muscle activity differences during walking', *Gait & Posture* 42(3), September 2015, https://www.sciencedirect.com/science/article/pii/S0966636215004993, last accessed on 6 February 2023.

13. Sadi Khan, 'The Truth About Arch Support – A Meta Analysis of 150 Studies', RunRepeat, 6 August 2021, https://runrepeat.com/arch-support-study, last accessed on 6 February 2023.

14. Sahar Ahmed Abdalbary, 'Foot Mobilization and Exercise Program Combined with Toe Separator Improves Outcomes in Women with Moderate Hallux Valgus at 1-Year Follow-up', *Journal of the American Podiatric Medical Association*, 108(6): 478-486, November 2018, https://pubmed.ncbi.nlm.nih.gov/29683337/, last accessed on 6 February 2023.

15. Kellie C. Huxel Bliven and Barton E. Anderson, 'Core Stability Training for Injury Prevention', *Sports Health*, 5(6): 514–22, November 2013, https://www.ncbi.nlm.nih.gov/pmc/articles/PMC3806175/, last accessed on 6 February 2023.

16. Guna Sankar, et al., 'Prevalence of low back pain and its relation to quality of life and disability among women in rural area of Puducherry, India', *Indian Journal of Pain*, 30(2): 111–15, 18 July 2016, https://indianjpain.org/article.asp?issn=0970-5333;year=2016;volume=30;issue=2;spage=111;epage=115;aulast=Ahdhi, last accessed on 6 February 2023.

17. Sushmi Dey, 'Knee implants to cost up to 69% less as government caps prices', *Times of India*, 25 September 2019, https://timesofindia.indiatimes.com/india/knee-implants-to-cost-up-to-69-less-as-government-caps-prices/articleshow/60094167.cms, last accessed on 6 February 2023.

18. Jawahir A Pachore, et al., 'ISHKS joint registry: A preliminary report', *Indian Journal of Orthopaedics*, 47(5): 505–09,

September–October 2013, https://www.ncbi.nlm.nih.gov/pmc/articles/PMC3796925/, last accessed on 6 February 2023.

19. Zhihong Zhao, et al., 'Static Low-Angle Squatting Reduces the Intra-Articular Inflammatory Cytokines and Improves the Performance of Patients with Knee Osteoarthritis', *BioMed Research International*, 30 October 2019, https://www.ncbi.nlm.nih.gov/pmc/articles/PMC6874930/, last accessed on 6 February 2023.

20. Emily Gersema, 'Squatting and kneeling may be better for your health than sitting', *University of Southern California News*, 9 March 2020, https://news.usc.edu/166572/squatting-kneeling-health-sitting-usc-research/, last accessed on 6 February 2023.

21. Bahram Jam, 'Deep squatting: Good or Bad?', *ResearchGate*, July 2015, https://www.researchgate.net/publication/306372512_Deep_squatting_Good_or_Bad, last accessed on 6 February 2023.

22. Matthew Kritz, et al., 'The Bodyweight Squat: A Movement Screen for the Squat Pattern', *Strength and Conditioning Journal*, 31(1):76–85, February 2009, https://www.researchgate.net/publication/232208909_The_Bodyweight_Squat_A_Movement_Screen_for_the_Squat_Pattern, last accessed on 6 February 2023.

23. Donald D. Harrison, et al., 'Sitting Biomechanics, Part II: Optimal Car Driver[apos]s Seat and Optimal Driver[apos]s Spinal Model, *Journal of Manipulative and Physiological Therapeutics*, 23(1): 37–47, February 2000, https://www.researchgate.net/publication/12655743_Sitting_Biomechanics_Part_II_Optimal_Car_Driverapos_s_Seat_and_Optimal_Driverapos_s_Spinal_Model, last accessed on 6 February 2023.

24. Lindsay J. Distefano, et al., 'Evidence Supporting Balance Training in Healthy Individuals: A Systemic Review', *Journal of Strength and Conditioning Research*, 23(9): 2718–31, November 2009, https://www.researchgate.net/publication/38086914_

Evidence_Supporting_Balance_Training_in_Healthy_
Individuals_A_Systemic_Review, last accessed on 6 February
2023.

25. Amanda Marchini, et al., 'Mixed Modal Training to Help Older
Adults Maintain Postural Balance', *Journal of Chiropractic
Medicine*, 18(3): 198–204, September 2019, https://www.
researchgate.net/publication/343806714_Mixed_Modal_
Training_to_Help_Older_Adults_Maintain_Postural_
Balance, last accessed on 6 February 2023.

26. Seung-Min Baik, et al., 'Understanding and Exercise of Gluteus
Medius Weakness: A Systematic Review', *Physical Therapy
Korea*, 28(1): 27–35, February 2021, https://www.researchgate.
net/publication/349465183_Understanding_and_Exercise_
of_Gluteus_Medius_Weakness_A_Systematic_Review, last
accessed on 6 February 2023.

27. Beom-Ryong Kim, et al., 'Effect of postural change on shoulder
joint internal and external rotation range of motion in healthy
adults in their 20's', *Physical Therapy Rehabilitation Science*,
30 September 2019, 8: 152–57, https://www.jptrs.org/journal/
view.html?doi=10.14474/ptrs.2019.8.3.152, last accessed on 6
February 2023.

28. Tae-Woon Kim, et al., 'Effects of elastic band exercise on
subjects with rounded shoulder posture and forward head
posture', *Journal of Physical Therapy Science*, 28 June 2016,
28(6): 1733–37, https://www.ncbi.nlm.nih.gov/pmc/articles/
PMC4932046/, last accessed on 6 February 2023.

29. Sam Ho-Park, et al., 'Effects of Lower Trapezius Strengthening
Exercises on Pain, Dysfunction, Posture Alignment, Muscle
Thickness and Contraction Rate in Patients with Neck
Pain', *Medical Science Monitor*, 26: e920208-1–e920208-
9, 2020, https://www.ncbi.nlm.nih.gov/pmc/articles/
PMC7115121/#:~:text=Conclusions,of%20the%20lower%20
trapezius%20muscle, last accessed on 6 February 2023.

30. Haifah Nitayarak and Pornpimol Charntaraviroj, 'Effects of scapular stabilization exercises on posture and muscle imbalances in women with upper crossed syndrome', *Journal of Back and Musculoskeletal Rehabilitation*, 34(3): 1–10, June 2021, https://www.researchgate.net/publication/352532595_Effects_of_scapular_stabilization_exercises_on_posture_and_muscle_imbalances_in_women_with_upper_crossed_syndrome_A_randomized_controlled_trial, last accessed on 6 February 2023.

31. Marc-Olivier Dubé, et al., 'Rotator cuff-related shoulder pain: Does the type of exercise influence the outcomes?', *BMJ Open*, 10(11): e039976, 2020, https://www.ncbi.nlm.nih.gov/pmc/articles/PMC7646354/, last accessed on 6 February 2023.

32. C. Lockard Conley and Robert S. Schwartz, 'Functions of blood', *Britannica*, https://www.britannica.com/science/blood-biochemistry/Platelets-thrombocytes, last accessed on 6 February 2023.

33. 'Unwinding the Mystery of Fascia', *Phys-Ed*, http://www.physednm.com/fascia/#:~:text=Fascia%20is%20composed%20mostly%20of,system%20to%20keep%20it%20supple, last accessed on 6 February 2023.

34. Serena Scarpelli, et al., 'The Functional Role of Dreaming in Emotional Processes, Project: Neurobiological bases of dream recall', *Frontiers in Psychology*, 10: 459, March 2019, https://www.researchgate.net/publication/331777904_The_Functional_Role_of_Dreaming_in_Emotional_Processes, last accessed on 6 February 2023.

35. C. Grippaudo, et al., 'Association between oral habits, mouth breathing and malocclusion', ACTA Otorhinolaryngologica Italia, 36(5): 386–94, October 2016, https://pubmed.ncbi.nlm.nih.gov/27958599/, last accessed on 6 February 2023.

36. 'Globalization of food systems in developing countries: impact on food security and nutrition', FAO, Food and nutrition paper

83, https://www.fao.org/3/y5736e/y5736e.pdf, last accessed on 6 February 2023.

37. Lesley M. Butler, et al., 'Prospective Study of Dietary Patterns and Persistent Cough with Phlegm among Chinese Singaporeans', *American Journal of Respiratory and Critical Care Medicine*, 173(3): 264–70, 1 February 2006, https://www.ncbi.nlm.nih.gov/pmc/articles/PMC1447591/, last accessed on 6 February 2023.

38. Sophie Svensson, et al., 'Increased net water loss by oral compared to nasal expiration in healthy subjects', *Rhinology* 44(1): 74–77, March 2006, https://pubmed.ncbi.nlm.nih.gov/16550955/, last accessed on 6 February 2023.

39. Dr Suresh Gowda, 'Sleep apnoea among kids: Things to know', *Indian Express*, 5 June 2022, https://indianexpress.com/article/parenting/health-fitness/sleep-apnea-among-kids-7595235/, last accessed on 6 February 2023.

40. 'Overeating impairs brain insulin function, a mechanism that can lead to diabetes and obesity', *Science Daily*, 17 October 2012, https://www.sciencedaily.com/releases/2012/10/121017153911.htm, last accessed on 6 February 2023.

41. Dinesh Thangavel, et al., 'Effect of 12 weeks of slow breathing exercise practice on anthropometric parameters in healthy volunteers', *National Journal of Physiology Pharmacy and Pharmacology*, 8(12): 1–5, October 2018, https://www.researchgate.net/publication/328189915_Effect_of_12_weeks_of_slow_breathing_exercise_practice_on_anthropometric_parameters_in_healthy_volunteers, last accessed on 6 February 2023.

42. Patrick McKeown, 'Part 111: The secret of Health 9. Rapid weight loss without dieting', *Oxygen Advantage*, William Morrow Paperbacks, 2016.

43. Ibid.

Chapter 4: What Is My Relationship with Pain?

1. Dirk De Ridder, et al., 'The anatomy of pain and suffering in the brain and its clinical implications', *Neuroscience & Bio behavioural Reviews*, 130: 125–46, https://www.sciencedirect.com/science/article/pii/S0149763421003560, last accessed on 6 February 2023.

2. Leslie J. Crofford, 'Chronic Pain: Where the Body Meets the Brain', *Transactions of the Amical Clinical and Climatological Association*, 126: 167–183, 2015, https://www.ncbi.nlm.nih.gov/pmc/articles/PMC4530716/, last accessed on 6 February 2023.

3. Micheal J. Shea, 'Chapter 16 – The Psychology of pain in musculoskeletal dysfunction', *Myofascial Release Therapy*, North Atlantic Books, 2014.

4. Karoline Cheung, et al., 'Delayed onset muscle soreness: Treatment strategies and performance factors', *Sports Med*, 33(2): 145–64, 2003, https://pubmed.ncbi.nlm.nih.gov/12617692/, last accessed on 6 February 2023.

5. Zachary Legault, et al. 'The Influence of Oral L-Glutamine Supplementation on Muscle Strength Recovery and Soreness Following Unilateral Knee Extension Eccentric Exercise', *International Journal of Sport Nutrition and Exercise Metabolism*, 25(5): 417–26, 2015.

6. Jan Dommerholt, et al., 'Myofascial Trigger Points: An Evidence-Informed Review', *Journal of Manual & Manipulative Therapy*, 14(4): 203–21, October 2006, https://www.researchgate.net/publication/233680399_Myofascial_Trigger_Points_An_Evidence-Informed_Review, last accessed on 6 February 2023.

7. 'IASP announces revised definition of pain', IASP News, 16 July 2020, https://www.iasp-pain.org/publications/iasp-news/iasp-announces-revised-definition-of-pain/, last accessed on 6 February 2023.

Chapter 5: Most Common Reasons for Pain

1. *Front Psychiatry*, 1(131), 24 September 2010.
2. Natalie A. Masento, et al., 'Effects of hydration status on cognitive performance and mood', *British Journal of Nutrition*, 111(10), Cambridge University Press, 30 January 2014, https://www.cambridge.org/core/journals/british-journal-of-nutrition/article/effects-of-hydration-status-on-cognitive-performance-and-mood/1210B6BE585E03C71A299C52B51B22F7, last accessed on 6 February 2023.
3. Chloe Bennett, 'How Does Mild Dehydration Affect the Body?', *News Medical Life Science*, 5 July 2019, https://www.news-medical.net/health/How-Does-Mild-Dehydration-Affect-the-Body.aspx, last accessed on 6 February 2023.
4. Sharon Kleyne, 'Air Conditioning Can Dehydrate Skin And Eyes, Reports Water and Health Researcher Sharon Kleyne', *Cision PRWeb*, 6 June 2022, https://www.prweb.com/releases/2013/7/prweb10962898.htm, last accessed on 6 February 2023.
5. Victor A. C. Lincoln, 'Effect of Dehydration in the UV Transmittance of "in vitro" Corneas', *Proceedings of SPIE - The International Society for Optical Engineering* 8209: 14, Research Gate, February 2012, https://www.researchgate.net/publication/258710852_Effect_of_Dehydration_in_the_UV_Transmittance_of_in_vitro_Corneas, last accessed on 6 February 2023.
6. Joseph M Donnelly, et al., 'Perpetuating Factors for Myofascial pain syndrome', *Travell, Simons and Simons' Myofascial Pain and Dysfunction—The Trigger Point Manual*, Walters Kluwer, 2019.
7. Natalie C. Ward, et al., 'Statin Toxicity' , *AHA Journal*, 124 (2): 328–350, 17 January 2019, https://doi.org/10.1161/CIRCRESAHA.118.312782.

8. Joon-Hee Lee, 'Effects of forward head posture on static and dynamic balance control', *Journal of Physical Therapy Science*, 28(1): 274–77, 2016, https://www.jstage.jst.go.jp/article/jpts/28/1/28_jpts-2015-702/_article, last accessed on 6 February 2023.

Chapter 6: Soft-Tissue Release to Fix Common Aches and Pains

1. Babak Missaghi, 'Sternocleidomastoid syndrome: A case study', *Journal of the Canadian Chiropractic Association*, 48(3): 201–05, September 2004, https://www.ncbi.nlm.nih.gov/pmc/articles/PMC1769463/, last accessed on 6 February 2023.
2. A. Karan, et al., 'A neglected reason of vertigo and a new approach to the patient with vertigo: Myofascial pain syndrome', *ResearchGate*, January 2008, https://www.researchgate.net/publication/297833828_A_neglected_reason_of_vertigo_and_a_new_approach_to_the_patient_with_vertigo_Myofascial_pain_syndrome, last accessed on 6 February 2023.
3. Dae Kyung Cho, et al., 'Myofascial Pain Syndrome in Patients with Cervical Vertigo', *Journal of Korean Academy of Rehabilitation Medicine*, 35: 243–49, 2011, https://www.e-arm.org/upload/pdf/Jkarm035-02-12.pdf, last accessed on 6 February 2023.
4. Carina A. C. Bezerra Rocha Tanit Ganz Sanchez, 'Myofascial Trigger Points: Occurrence and Capacity to Modulate Tinnitus Perception', *International Archives of Otorhinolaryngology*, 10(3), July/September 2006.
5. Rodrigo Lorenzi Poluha, et al., 'Myofascial trigger points in patients with temporomandibular joint disc displacement with reduction: a cross-sectional study', *Journal of Applied Oral Science*, 26: e20170578, May 2018, https://www.ncbi.nlm.nih.

gov/pmc/articles/PMC6010330/, last accessed on 6 February 2023.

6. Thien Phu Do, et al., 'Myofascial trigger points in migraine and tension-type headache', *The Journal of Headache and Pain*, 19, Article no: 84, 2018, https://thejournalofheadacheandpain. biomedcentral.com/articles/10.1186/s10194-018-0913-8, last accessed on 6 February 2023.

7. Babak Missaghi, 'Sternocleidomastoid syndrome: a case study', *Journal of the Canadian Chiropractic Association*, 48(3): 201–05, September 2004, https://www.ncbi.nlm.nih. gov/pmc/articles/PMC1769463/, last accessed on 6 February 2023.

8. Ibid.

9. Gordon E. Lawson, et al, 'A case of pseudo–angina pectoris from a pectoralis minor trigger point caused by cross-country skiing', *Journal of Chiropractic Medicine*, 10(3): 173–78, September 2011, https://www.ncbi.nlm.nih.gov/pmc/articles/ PMC3259990/, last accessed on 6 February 2023.

10. Elizabeth Anne Pastore and Wendy B. Katzman, 'Recognizing Myofascial Pelvic Pain in the Female Patient with Chronic Pelvic Pain', *Journal of Obstetric, Gynecologic, & Neonatal Nursing*, 41(5): 680–91, 3 August 2012, https://pubmed.ncbi. nlm.nih.gov/22862153/, last accessed on 6 February 2023.

11. Muhammad Kashif, et al., 'Association of myofascial trigger points in neck and shoulder region with depression, anxiety and stress among university students', *Journal Of Pakistan Medical Association*, 71(9): 2139–42, September 2021, https:// pubmed.ncbi.nlm.nih.gov/34580502/, last accessed on 6 February 2023.

12. Stephen E. Epstein, et al., 'Chest wall syndrome, a common cause of unexplained cardiac pain', *JAMA Network*, 241:2793– 97, 1979, https://jamanetwork.com/journals/jama/article-abstract/365484, last accessed on 6 February 2023.

Chapter 8: Movement and Mental Health

1. Ashish Sharma, et al., 'Exercise for Mental Health', *Primary Care Companion to the Journal of Clinical Psychiatry*, 8(2): 106, 2006, https://www.ncbi.nlm.nih.gov/pmc/articles/PMC1470658/, last accessed on 6 February 2023.

2. Bruce A. Watkins, 'Endocannabinoids, exercise, pain, and a path to health with aging', *Molecular Aspects of Medicine*, 64: 68–78, 5 October 2018, https://pubmed.ncbi.nlm.nih.gov/30290200/, last accessed on 6 February 2023.

3. Yongsoon Park and Bruce A. Watkins, 'Vitamins and Hormones, 2021, Endocannabinoids and aging-Inflammation, neuroplasticity, mood and pain', *Vitamins and Hormones*, 129–72, 29 January 2021, https://pubmed.ncbi.nlm.nih.gov/33706946/, last accessed on 6 February 2023.

4. Bruce A. Watkins, 'Diet, endocannabinoids, and health', *Nutrition Research New York*, 70: 32–39, October 2019, https://pubmed.ncbi.nlm.nih.gov/31280882/, last accessed on 6 February 2023.

5. O'Llenecia S. Walker, et al., 'The role of the endocannabinoid system in female reproductive tissues', *Journal of Ovarian Research*, 12(1), January 2019, https://pubmed.ncbi.nlm.nih.gov/30646937/, last accessed on 6 February 2023.

6. Maria Morena, et al., 'Neurobiological Interactions between Stress and the Endocannabinoid System', *Neuropsychopharmacology*, 41(1): 80–102, January 2016, https://www.nature.com/articles/npp2015166, last accessed on 6 February 2023.

7. Emma L. Scotter, et al., 'The endocannabinoid system as a target for the treatment of neurodegenerative disease', *British Journal of Pharmacology*, 160(3): 480–98, June 2010, https://www.ncbi.nlm.nih.gov/pmc/articles/PMC2931550/, last accessed on 6 February 2023.

8.   Paul D. Loprinzi, 'The Endocannabinoid System as a Potential Mechanism through which Exercise Influences Episodic Memory Function', *Brain Science*, 9(5): 112, 9 May 2019, https://www.ncbi.nlm.nih.gov/pmc/articles/PMC6562547/, last accessed on 6 February 2023.

9.   David, J, Lindin, 'The Truth Behind "Runner's High" and Other Mental Benefits of Running', *John Hopkins Medicine*, https://www.hopkinsmedicine.org/health/wellness-and-prevention/the-truth-behind-runners-high-and-other-mental-benefits-of-running, last accessed on 6 February 2023.

10. David A. Raichlen, et al., 'Exercise-induced endocannabinoid signalling is modulated by intensity', Raichlen Arizona, (2012), *European Journal of Applied Physiology*, 113: 869–75, 2013, http://www.raichlen.arizona.edu/DavePDF/RaichlenEtAl2013.pdf, last accessed on 6 February 2023.

11. Oliver Stoll, et al., 'Peak Performance, the Runner's High and Flow', ResearchGate, Project: Psychological aspects of running and ultra-running, November 2018, in *Handbook of Sports and Exercise Psychology*, ed. Mark Anshel, American Psychology Association (APA), https://www.researchgate.net/publication/317568272_Peak_Performance_the_Runner's_High_and_Flow, last accessed on 6 February 2023.

12. *Journal of Personality and Social Psychology* 92(6): 1087–101, July 2007.

13. Anna Katharina Schaffner, 'Perseverance in psychology: 4 activities to improve perseverance', *Positive Psychology*, 6 September 2020, https://www.annakschaffner.com/post/perseverance-in-psychology-4-activities-to-improve-perseverance, last accessed on 6 February 2023.

14. Wikipedia, 'Neurobiological effects of physical exercise', https://en.m.wikipedia.org/wiki/Neurobiological_effects_of_physical_exercise, last accessed on 6 February 2023.

15. Oliver Stoll, et al., 'Peak Performance, the Runner's High and Flow', *ResearchGate*, Project: Psychological aspects of running and ultra-running, November 2018, in *Handbook of Sports and Exercise Psychology*, ed. Mark Anshel, American Psychology Association (APA), https://www.researchgate.net/publication/317568272_Peak_Performance_the_Runner's_High_and_Flow, last accessed on 6 February 2023.

Scan QR code to access the
Penguin Random House India website